# PROFILES OF THE NUTRIENTS

## 2. MINERALS AND TRACE ELEMENTS

# PROFILES OF THE NUTRIENTS

## 2. Minerals and Trace Elements

## RICHARD RYDON

## Non-fiction

First Paperback Edition: January 2017

ISBN: 978-1-326-88675-2

Cover image – ID 7499030 – tonobalaguer/123RF.com

# Contents

# Preface

This series of three books includes an account of the nutrients known to be essential for human life. Appropriately, the text is called PROFILES OF THE NUTRIENTS. The series covers some fifty different nutrients. It is intended primarily as an outline for those who seek an introduction to the nutrients presented in a direct way.

The classical definition of a nutrient is an essential substance in food that provides structural or functional components or energy to the body. The ability to provide energy requires one other essential substance that does not come from food, namely oxygen gas.

There are no value judgements on the special merits of selected nutrients. All are equally essential for human life. Each nutrient is identified in the text by:

- A Chapter of its own
- Common name and alternative names
- Some key historical dates (e.g. for the discovery of the vitamins)
- The Nature of each nutrient
- Biological functions
- Daily requirement and food sources
- Toxicity symptoms
- Deficiency symptoms

Book 1 considers carbohydrate, lipid and protein, book 2 considers minerals and trace elements and book 3 considers vitamins. Overall, the series presents a concise outline of each of the essential nutrients.

# 29

## Body Composition and the Elements

The six major elements in the human body are listed in Table 29.1.

- Most of the oxygen is combined with hydrogen in the form of water.

- Most of the remaining oxygen and hydrogen is combined with carbon in the form of carbohydrate, lipid and protein.

- Nitrogen occurs in amino acids, proteins and nucleic acids and in some complex carbohydrates and porphyrins.

  These elements are rarely considered individually but only insofar as they comprise essential nutrients.

- About 17 percent of the phosphorous in the body occurs organically bound in phospholipids, phosphoproteins and nucleic acids and many intermediate compounds. The remaining 83 percent occurs as inorganic phosphate and about 80 percent of this occurs in the bones and teeth. In this form, it is best considered as a mineral (see Chapter 33). Inorganic phosphate is combined with oxygen and hydrogen and may be denoted as $P_i$ for short. Phosphate expressed as total inorganic phosphate includes two anionic forms, $H_2PO_4^-$ and $HPO_4^{2-}$. Acidic environments favour the $H_2PO_4^-$ form. Inorganic phosphate comprises one of the six major minerals in the human body, as illustrated in Table 29.2.

- Sulphur occurs in proteins in the form of sulphur-containing amino acids (such as cysteine and methionine) and traces also occur in some complex carbohydrates such as chondroitin sulphates. More than half the sulphate in the body comes from metabolism of these compounds. The remainder occurs as inorganic sulphate, $SO_4^{2-}$, which is the form required for the synthesis of 3'-phosphoadenosine-5'-phosphosulphate, a compound known as active sulphate. A deficiency of sulphate is not found in people who consume normal protein intakes which contain sufficient sulphur-containing amino acids. High intake levels of inorganic sulphate may cause diarrhoea.

The abovementioned elements, together with the six major minerals, namely calcium, phosphorous, potassium, sodium, chloride and magnesium, account for 99.9 percent of the mass of the human body. Not all the elements making up the remaining 0.1 percent are biologically essential. Important trace elements, necessary for mammalian life, include iron, cobalt, copper, zinc, manganese, molybdenum, iodine, and selenium. Only about one quarter of all the elements in the periodic table are known to have biological functions. Of the remainder, some are highly toxic, some are relatively non-toxic and some are solely considered of therapeutic interest.

So, of the hundred or so different elements found in nature, only eleven are of major occurrence in the human body, and only another ten or so, which occur in smaller amounts, are generally accepted as essential elements. These are listed in Tables 29.1, 29.2 and 29.3.

An analyst could arguably conclude that only about 5 grams out of a total of 70,000 grams of the human body is not essential. In contrast with the relative abundance in the body, Table 29.4 summarises the relative daily requirements for the known essential minerals and trace elements in humans. The following chapters in this book are presented in the same sequence of (approximately) decreasing daily intake needs.

Some additional elements, many of which do not yet generally qualify as nutrients for humans, are considered in Chapter 45. Tables 29.5 and 29.6, include these, comparing their occurrence in the body and their typical daily intakes by humans. Some of these have associated deficiency symptoms in plants and animals but do not have any known biological role. Until recently, bromide had no known biochemical function in humans. Some forms of an element,

2

such as chromium, are highly toxic in minute doses but other forms of the same element may still be essential. Several minerals which are not necessary for mammals, may be necessary for various other forms of life. The total number of elements that are essentially needed for any organism is not definitively known and so is subject to revision.

**Table 29.1.** The major elements stored in the body

| Element | Symbol | Approximate amount (kilograms) |
|---|---|---|
| Oxygen | O | 45.8 |
| Carbon | C | 12.6 |
| Hydrogen | H | 7.0 |
| Nitrogen | N | 2.1 |
| Phosphorous | P | 0.8 |
| Sulphur | S | 0.2 |

Total body weight is taken to be 70 kg.
The phosphorous value includes the inorganic forms.

**Table 29.2.** The major minerals stored in the body

| Mineral | Symbol | Approximate amount (grams) |
|---|---|---|
| Calcium | $Ca^{2+}$ | 1,100 |
| Inorganic Phosphate | $P_i$ | 650 |
| Potassium | $K^+$ | 140 |
| Sodium | $Na^+$ | 105 |
| Chloride | $Cl^-$ | 105 |
| Magnesium | $Mg^{2+}$ | 35 |

The symbol K for potassium is taken from the Latin *kalium*. The symbol Na for sodium is taken from the Latin *natrium*.

The above listed six minerals are occasionally referred to as macroelements. The term macroelement includes minerals and nonminerals. So, some authors include inorganic sulphate in this table.

**Table 29.3.** The essential minerals, trace and ultratrace elements stored in the body

| Element | Symbol | Approximate amount (milligrams) |
|---|---|---|
| Calcium | $Ca^{2+}$ | 1,100,000 |
| Phosphate | $P_i$ | 650,000 |
| Potassium | $K^+$ | 140,000 |
| Sodium | $Na^+$ | 105,000 |
| Chloride | $Cl^-$ | 105,000 |
| Magnesium | $Mg^{2+}$ | 35,000 |
| Iron | Fe | 4,000 |
| Zinc | Zn | 2,300 |
| Fluoride | $F^-$ | 2,000 |
| Copper | Cu | 100 |
| Iodine | I | 20 |
| Selenium | Se | 15 |
| Chromium | Cr | 14 |
| Manganese | Mn | 12 |
| Molybdenum | Mo | 5 |
| Cobalt | Co | 3 |

The absolute quantity of each element in the body is highly variable. Therefore, the sequence above, which is given in approximately descending order of abundance, is liable to some variation from person to person. The symbols for the elements are obvious except for tin; Sn is taken from the Latin stannous.

Some of the above are occasionally referred to as microelements rather than trace elements.

**Table 29.4.** Daily requirement for the essential minerals, trace and ultratrace elements

| NAME | RELATIVE ADULT REQUIREMENT (micrograms per day) | |
|---|---|---|
| | Male | Female |
| *Minerals* | | |
| Potassium | 4,700,000 | 4.700,000 |
| Chloride | 2,300,000 | 2,300,000 |
| Sodium | 1,500,000 | 1,500,000 |
| Calcium | 1,000,000 | 1,000,000 |
| Phosphorous | 700,000 | 700,000 |
| Magnesium | 420,000 | 320,000 |
| *Trace Elements* | | |
| Iron | 8,000 | 18,000 |
| Zinc | 11,000 | 8,000 |
| Fluoride | 4,000 | 3,000 |
| Manganese | 2,300 | 1,800 |
| *Ultratrace Elements* | | |
| Copper | 900 | 900 |
| Iodine | 150 | 150 |
| Selenium | 55 | 55 |
| Molybdenum | 45 | 45 |
| Chromium | 35 | 25 |
| Cobalt (as $B_{12}$) | (0.1) | (0.1) |

The daily requirements given are approximate. Minerals and trace elements will be considered in the above order in the following chapters. Cobalt, however, is considered in Part 3, in the chapter on vitamin $B_{12}$.

There is no absolute distinction between minerals, trace elements and ultratrace elements other than the relative amounts of them required or ingested per day where, generally, the amounts are grams, milligrams and micrograms respectively.

**Table 29.5.** Trace and ultratrace elements stored in the body

| Element | Symbol | Approximate amount (milligrams) |
| --- | --- | --- |
| Iron | Fe | 4,000 |
| Fluoride | F | 2,600 |
| Zinc | Zn | 2,300 |
| Silicon | Si | 1,000 |
| Rubidium | Rb | 680 |
| Strontium | Sr | 320 |
| Bromide | Br | 260 |
| Lead | Pb | 120 |
| Copper | Cu | 70 |
| Aluminium | Al | 60 |
| Cadmium | Cd | 50 |
| Barium | Ba | 22 |
| Iodine | I | 20 |
| Tin | Sn | 20 |
| Boron | B | 18 |
| Selenium | Se | 15 |
| Nickel | Ni | 15 |
| Manganese | Mn | 12 |
| Chromium | Cr | 14 |
| Arsenic | As | 7 |
| Lithium | Li | 7 |
| Molybdenum | Mo | 5 |
| Germanium | Ge | 5 |
| Cobalt | Co | 3 |
| Silver | Ag | 2 |
| Gold | Au | 0.2 |
| Vanadium | V | 0.1 |

Not all of these elements are considered essential in humans.

The absolute quantity of each element in the body is highly variable. Therefore, the sequence above, which is given in approximately descending order of abundance, is liable to some variation from person to person. The symbols for the elements are obvious except for tin; Sn is taken from the Latin stannous.

**Table 29.6.** Suggested or typical daily requirements or
intakes for trace and ultratrace elements

| NAME | Typical adult daily intakes or amounts possibly required (micrograms per day) |
|---|---|
| Tin | 1,000 – 40,000 |
| Silicon | 2,000 – 35,000 |
| Iron * | 8,000 – 18,000 |
| Boron | 1,000 – 13,000 |
| Zinc * | 8,000 – 11,000 |
| Aluminium | 2,000 – 10,000 |
| Bromide | 2,000 – 8,000 |
| Rubidium | 1,000 – 5,000 |
| Strontium | 1,000 – 5,000 |
| Fluoride * | 3,000 – 4,000 |
| Manganese * | 1,800 – 2,300 |
| Barium | 440 – 1,800 |
| Germanium | 400 – 1,500 |
| Copper * | 900 – 1,300 |
| Lithium | 200 – 600 |
| Iodine * | 150 – 290 |
| Nickel | 25 – 260 |
| Lead | 15 – 100 |
| Silver | 30 – 90 |
| Selenium * | 55 – 70 |
| Molybdenum * | 45 – 50 |
| Chromium * | 25 – 35 |
| Arsenic | 12 – 25 |
| Cadmium | 10 – 20 |
| Vanadium | 10 – 15 |
| Cobalt (as $B_{12}$) * | (0.1) |
| Gold | 0.01 – 0.1 |

* These essential nutrients have established daily requirements

# 30

# POTASSIUM

## Common Name

Potassium (elemental), (K).

## Alternative Names

*Kalium, Kali.*
Potassium ion ($K^+$).
Potash.
Mineral. Electrolyte.

## Nature

Potassium is classified as an alkali metal in the s-block, group 1 (IA), period 4, of the periodic table of elements. It exists as the monovalent potassium cation $K^+$. This is the only form of interest as far as nutrition is concerned. Hence potassium is one of the major electrolytes in the body. Other members in the group include lithium Li, sodium Na, and rubidium Rb, and in many respects, even hydrogen H, may be considered to fall into this group. The symbol for potassium, K, comes from the Latin word *kalium*.

## Biological Functions

- Potassium is positively charged. Each potassium ion carries one positive charge. Therefore, potassium contributes significantly to the electrolyte content of the cell.

- In general, about sixty percent of the body water is inside the cells. And potassium is the main cation found in the intracellular fluid. In contrast, sodium is the main cation found in the extracellular fluid.

- Potassium, together with sodium, is involved in the transmission of nerve impulses. In this context, the exact ratios of the ions across the membranes determines the cell surface charge or membrane potential.

- Maintaining the correct ratio of potassium to sodium across the cell membranes is essential, especially for muscle and nerve cells.

- The ratio of potassium to sodium is also essential for proper fluid balance in the body, with potassium tending to decrease the water load and sodium tending to increase it. One of the chief functions of potassium is to maintain the correct osmolality (osmotic pressure) inside the cells.

- Potassium serves to maintain the acid-base balance in the body because of its ability to exchange for hydrogen ions which are the acid-producing ions in the body. The kidney tends to reabsorb potassium in exchange for hydrogen ions which are thus eliminated in the urine.

- Potassium influences the activity of several enzymes involved in various processes such as energy and carbohydrate metabolism and protein synthesis. The following enzymes require potassium for their action

  Sodium, potassium-ATPase which breaks down ATP releasing energy to drive other chemical reactions

  Pyruvate kinase which is involved in glycolysis

  Dimethylmalate dehydrogenase which is an oxidoreductase enzyme

  2-Isopropylmalate synthase which is a transferase enzyme

  (R)-Aminopropanol dehydrogenase which is involved in glycine, serine and threonine metabolism

  Tryptophanase which converts L-tryptophan to pyruvate

- Potassium has an irritant effect on certain tissues such as muscle cells. This effect like that of sodium is counteracted by calcium.

## Requirement

The typical Western diet provides some 2 to 5 grams of potassium per day. It is important to keep the correct balance between potassium and sodium intake. If sodium intake is increased abnormally then the requirement for potassium also increases. Unfortunately, additional sodium salt is invariably added to food either directly or during processing, so the recommended intake values for potassium reflect this requirement. Potassium is widely distributed and although it is easy to measure, food values are highly variable. But even though there is considerable variation in certain foodstuffs, nevertheless the average intake of potassium is always sufficient to prevent deficiency in healthy individuals. Two grams of potassium or more are lost in the urine per day in a typical adult. Most of the potassium in the diet occurs in plant foods such as fruit and vegetables. A potassium compendium is included in Table 30.1. **The recommended adult daily intake of potassium in both males and in females is 4.7 g/d.** Potassium is readily absorbed mainly in the small intestine and does not require an active transport mechanism.

## Toxicity

Potassium toxicity is termed hyperkalemia. Prolonged intake of some potassium supplements may increase the risk of ulceration of the stomach. On the other hand, potassium salt when used as a substitute for sodium salt (the common table salt) does not cause irritation of the gut. A sudden excessive buildup of potassium in the blood (by intravenous infusion) may cause the heart to stop beating in diastole, but this does not occur as a result of oral intakes from food. Toxicity is likely to arise if the intake of potassium exceeds 25 grams per day. This level overloads the ability of the kidneys to remove excess potassium. Severe potassium toxicity may result following kidney failure or a decrease in the hormones of the adrenal cortex. After severe injury or burns potassium may leak out of the cells into the blood. This is one complication of shock.

# Deficiency

A deficiency of potassium is termed hypokalemia. A dietary deficiency of potassium in humans is extremely rare. Some conditions such as protein-energy malnutrition or prolonged treatment with diuretics or renal failure can however result in potassium depletion. Apart from diuretics, chronic use of laxatives may also cause potassium depletion. Diarrhoea itself produces the same effect if prolonged. During chronic depletion, the intracellular potassium may be used to keep the blood (extracellular) levels at a sufficient normal level. This complicates the diagnosis of deficiency. Also, if potassium is very low, the cells may begin to use hydrogen ions instead which results in an increased acidity thus causing a condition called intracellular acidosis. At the same time the kidneys also begin to excrete more hydrogen ions instead of the usual amount of potassium ions, and this produces the opposite effect in the blood namely, increased alkalinity which causes an extracellular alkalosis. Eventually the blood potassium level falls. Potassium deficiency results in a general muscular weakness and this may be accompanied by mental confusion. The condition is more common in the elderly, particularly if they are on certain medications. Further effects include a slowing of certain nerve and muscle reflexes, constipation and distension of the abdomen. The skin becomes dry in many cases. As with a severe potassium toxicity a gross deficiency of potassium may also cause heart attacks. In certain experimental animals, potassium depletion results in retarded growth and muscular paralysis. Other symptoms include enlargement of the heart and kidneys, low blood pressure, vomiting, coma and ultimately death.

**Table 30.1.** Potassium compendium

| FOOD GROUP | POTASSIUM LEVEL |
| --- | --- |
| Milk and products | Low |
| Eggs | Low |
| Meat and fish | Medium |
| Fats and oils | Nil |
| Grain and products | Medium |
| Nuts and pulses | Very high |
| Root vegetables | High |
| Leaf vegetables | High |
| Fruit | High |
| Sweets | Very low, variable |

Potassium values are very variable.

# 31

## CHLORIDE

### Common Name

Chloride ($Cl^-$).

### Alternative Names

*Mur.* (from muriatic acid now called hydrochloric acid, HCl).
Chlorine (elemental not gaseous), (Cl, not $Cl_2$).
Mineral. Electrolyte.

### Nature

Chlorine itself is classified as a nonmetal in the p-block, group 17 (VIIB), period 3, of the periodic table of elements. It is a member of the halogen group and it exists as the monovalent chloride anion $Cl^-$. This is the only form of interest in nutrition. Hence chloride is one of the major electrolytes in the body. Other members of the group include fluorine F, bromine Br, and iodine I. A diverse collection of biogenic organohalogens are produced by living organisms but, apart from iodine, are of uncertain nutritional significance in humans.

### Biological Functions

- Chloride is negatively charged, and each chloride caries one negative charge. Chloride contributes significantly to the electrolyte composition of blood plasma.

- Chloride is very closely associated with potassium and sodium. The overall level of chloride in the body tends to reflect the total level of potassium plus sodium.

- Chloride is found mainly in the fluid surrounding cells, alongside sodium. About 15% of chloride in the body is located inside cells, with the highest amounts in red blood cells. Traces of chloride are also present in bones.

- Together with potassium and sodium, chloride is involved in determining the cell surface charge or membrane potential which is critical for the proper functioning of muscle and nerve cells. In this context, chloride is an important anion involved in maintaining electrolyte balance across cell membranes.

- Like potassium and sodium, chloride is essentially involved in maintaining the osmolality in the body and keeping the amount of fluid within and around cells in balance. Together with sodium, it is chiefly involved in maintaining the osmotic pressure of the blood.

- Chloride helps regulate the pH (acid-base) balance of body fluids.

- Chloride has certain special functions of its own. For example, it is involved in the formation of gastric juice in the stomach, which is essentially pure hydrochloric acid (HCl) and is vital for maintaining the normal acidic environment needed by pepsin, and aids digestion and absorption of many nutrients including iron and vitamin $B_{12}$.

- Chloride, like sodium, has little effect on enzyme activity. However, there is some evidence that it may have a role to play with the starch-splitting enzyme called amylase found in saliva.

- In the blood, there is a constant exchange between the chloride ion and the bicarbonate ion. This exchange is called the chloride shift. What happens is an exchange between bicarbonate inside the red blood cells and chloride in the plasma outside the cells. Effectively, this increases the efficiency of carbon dioxide transport from the tissues and its exchange at the lungs.

# Requirement

Chloride intakes and requirements are closely linked with sodium. In adult diets, there is a direct relationship between chloride and sodium intake which parallels the ratio of the two ions in common table salt. In other words, every three grams of chloride are accompanied by two grams of sodium. Interestingly the proposed intakes reflect this ratio. The only exception occurs for very young infants where the ratio reflects the composition of human milk. The recommended adult daily intake of chloride in both males and in females is 2.3 g/d.

Because of the abovementioned link, chloride food tables are in many respects redundant, even though chloride is easy to measure. Nevertheless, a chloride compendium is included for reference (Table 31.1).

# Toxicity

Chloride is very closely associated with sodium and potassium in food and also in the body. Consequently, an excess of either sodium or potassium is almost invariably accompanied by a corresponding excess of chloride. Until recently it was believed that chloride itself was non-toxic. It was considered that only the increases in the companion ions produced the toxic symptoms. Recently it has been suggested that perhaps it is a high chloride rather than a high sodium which causes one form of high blood pressure. This theory is of great interest but remains to be proved. It has been suggested that chloride intakes in excess of 15 grams per day may cause a number of unpleasant side effects, including vomiting convulsions, respiratory distress, and ultimately death.

The ionic form of the element, namely chloride, is the only form of interest in nutrition. Another form of the element namely chlorine is occasionally added to tap water and swimming pools as a disinfectant. This form is of no nutritional value but may have adverse toxic effects in high concentrations. The main risk is that chlorine accelerates the breakdown of vitamin E. Also from the purely cosmetic point of view chlorine may damage the hair, and

17

therefore should be well rinsed out after swimming in indoor pools. Another risk of excess chlorine is that it may reduce the natural level of certain gut bacteria which are beneficial and contribute to the daily requirements of certain vitamins notably biotin and vitamin K.

## Deficiency

A deficiency of chloride is known as hypochloremia. In normal individuals, chloride is rarely deficient. However, prolonged bouts of vomiting or diarrhoea may significantly reduce the level of chloride in the body. Large amounts of chloride with sodium can be lost during heavy sweating. Other causes include overuse of diuretics, over-hydration, burns congestive heart failure, certain kidney disorders and Addison's disease. A deficiency of potassium or sodium is inevitably accompanied by a deficiency of chloride. Deficiency of chloride can lead to a loss of appetite, muscle weakness, dehydration and alkalosis resulting in a high blood pH. A local effect in the stomach leading to a lack of formation of gastric juice (a condition called achlorhydria) is not caused directly by chloride deficiency, but is a disease of certain stomach cells. Decreased levels of blood chloride are found in diabetic patients, and following certain fevers and pneumonia.

**Table 31.1.** Chloride compendium

| FOOD GROUP | CHLORIDE LEVEL |
|---|---|
| Milk / Products | Low / Very high, variable |
| Eggs | Low |
| Meat and fish | Very   variable |
| Fats / Oils | High, variable / Nil |
| Grain / Products | Very low / High, variable |
| Nuts and pulses | Low, variable |
| Root vegetables | Very low |
| Leaf vegetables | Very low |
| Fruit | Very low |
| Sweets | Nil, variable |

# 32

# SODIUM

## Common Name

Sodium (elemental), (Na).

## Alternative Names

*Natrium, Nat.*
Sodium ion ($Na^+$).
Table Salt (somewhat incorrectly).
Mineral. Electrolyte.

## Nature

Sodium is classified as an alkali metal in the s-block, group 1 (IA), period 3, of the periodic table of elements. It exists as the monovalent sodium cation $Na^+$. This is the only form of interest as far as nutrition is concerned. Hence sodium is one of the major electrolytes in the body. Other members in the group include lithium Li, potassium K, and rubidium Rb, and in many respects, even hydrogen H, may be considered to fall into this group. The symbol for sodium Na, comes from the Latin word *natrium*.

## Biological Functions

- Sodium is positively charged. Like potassium, each sodium carries one positive charge. But in contrast to potassium, sodium contributes significantly to the electrolyte content of the blood plasma rather than to the cell water.

- In general, about forty percent of the body water occurs outside the cells. sodium is the main cation found in extracellular fluid. In contrast, potassium is the main cation found in intracellular fluid.

- The ratio of sodium to potassium is also essential for proper fluid balance in the body, with sodium tending to increase the water load and potassium tending to decrease it. In fact, one of the chief functions of sodium is to maintain the correct osmolality (osmotic pressure) outside the cells and particularly in the blood.

- The correct ratio of sodium to potassium across the cell membrane is essential, especially for nerve and muscle cells. Sodium, together with potassium and chloride, determine the cell surface charge or membrane potential which is critical for certain muscle and nerve cells.

- Sodium is involved in the absorption of glucose and galactose from the gut. The hexose transporter involved is sodium-dependent This transports both sodium ions and glucose together into the enterocyte. The transporter first binds sodium on the lumen side of the gut. Glucose can then bind and both sodium and glucose are transported into the cell. Sodium then dissociates into the cytoplasm of the cell and then glucose can dissociate.

- Unlike potassium, sodium has little effect on the activity of enzymes in the body, although it is involved in regulating the energy-providing enzyme ATPase.

- Sodium in conjunction with bicarbonate helps to regulate the acid-base balance of the blood by mobilising hydrogen ions in a kidney mechanism.

## Requirement

Sodium intake is very closely linked with chloride. Common table salt is pure sodium chloride and every gram of salt contains some 400 milligrams of sodium and 600 milligrams of chloride. A total sodium chloride intake of 750 mg per day is sufficient to maintain the sodium balance. This amount is provided by a vegetarian diet without added salt. Intake rates anywhere from about 600 to 3,500 mg per day seem perfectly adequate in temperate climates. The recommended adult daily intake of sodium in both males and in females is 1.5 g/d.

Sweating dramatically increases the need for sodium. Anywhere from 2 to 7 grams of sodium may lost per litre of sweat. Average sodium intakes are considerably greater than the amount required in most circumstances. Intake levels of 10,000 to 29,000 mg per day are the norm in some places. Continuous high intakes of sodium may have adverse effects particularly in susceptible individuals and especially in infants. Sodium is readily absorbed from the gut and does not require an active transport mechanism. Sodium is widely distributed in food and is easy to measure. A sodium compendium is included here for reference (Table 32.1). Tinned vegetables, meat and fish, often contain significant amounts of added salt, thereby increasing the sodium chloride levels. A typical increase of 200 to 300 mg sodium and 300 to 450 mg chloride per 100 grams of food over normal values can be expected unless the product specifies that no salt has been added. Tomato sauce itself contains very high concentrations of sodium (around 1,000 mg) and chloride (around 1,800 mg) per 100 g. Excess salt is also added to nuts, crisps, savories and cornflakes. In addition, (or sometimes instead of) common salt, the sodium or potassium salts of phosphate are often added to processed foods thereby increasing these respective contents unexpectedly. As seen above, the average daily intake of sodium is 25 grams per day in places, with values up to 50 grams per day occasionally being reported. Ignoring these extremes, the usual levels of intake are in the range 3 to 20 grams per day with a typical average nearer 15 grams per day. Because of the possible link between high blood pressure and excessive sodium intake in certain individuals it is advisable to limit salt intakes. A level of about 6 grams per day can be easily achieved by avoiding distinctly salty foods and the use of table salt with meals. A level of about 3 grams per day can be achieved by avoiding sauces, cakes and biscuits (which can be deceptively rich in salt). But levels of 1 gram per day can only be achieved by restricting the diet to special foods or remaining on a vegetarian diet.

## Toxicity

Recklessly, the average intake of sodium in most diets is markedly greater than the value required to maintain balance. Even so, the kidneys rapidly adapt to this sodium overload by excreting excess sodium in the urine. A toxicity due to sodium is sometimes termed hypernatremia. One of the first symptoms is a feeling of thirst. There is a desire to drink but the formation of urine is decreased. Consequently, there occurs a retention of water. After a single salty meal, this fluid retention may last for several hours. Chronic water retention is a more serious condition that requires medical treatment.

Sodium may also irritate certain tissues such as muscle cells. The irritation is counteracted by calcium ions, but the mechanism of this effect is poorly understood. Excessive sodium is excreted by the kidneys and this process requires additional water. Normally about 2 grams of sodium are excreted per litre of urine. The main symptoms of regular excess sodium include oedema, high blood pressure, abnormal heart activity, enlarged heart and kidneys and nephritis. Recently it has been suggested that is the excess chloride that accompanies sodium rather than the sodium itself which may be primarily responsible for the high blood pressure effect. In practice this is merely splitting hairs as far as nutrition is concerned and in theory it will be very difficult to prove.

## Deficiency

A deficiency of sodium is sometimes termed hyponatremia but is very rare. The loss of as little as 10 grams of sodium from the body can result in marked deficiency symptoms. Normally there is a gross excess of sodium. Nevertheless, in hot climates or during any exercise which results in profuse sweating a deficiency can arise if the salt lost is not replaced. In such circumstances where the sodium is not replaced, there occurs a redistribution of sodium from within the cells to maintain the level in the blood at the normal level. Also, the kidneys tend to conserve sodium more efficiently. Chronic deficiency of sodium will cause a stunting of growth. In certain experimental animals, low sodium reduces appetite, slows growth and interferes with the proper metabolism of lipids, proteins and energy. There also occurs a concentration of the blood due to increased water loss and this results in the retention of urea. Other effects are an increased viscosity of the blood while at the same time an overall reduced blood pressure and a rapid heartbeat. There occurs a general dehydration, dryness of the mouth and mental confusion. If a large quantity of water is taken immediately after dehydration, water intoxication may result. It is important to replace the sodium lost to avoid this effect. The human kidneys can adapt to excrete salt (NaCl) anywhere in the range from as little as 1 gram to 40 grams per day depending on intake.

**Table 32.1.** Sodium compendium

| FOOD GROUP | SODIUM LEVEL |
| --- | --- |
| Milk / Products | Very low / Very high |
| Eggs | Low |
| Meat and fish | Very variable |
| Fats / Oils | High / Nil |
| Grain / Products | Nil / High |
| Nuts and pulses | Nil |
| Root vegetables | Very low |
| Leaf vegetables | Very low |
| Fruit | Nil |
| Sweets | Nil |

# 33

# CALCIUM

## Common Name

Calcium (elemental), (Ca).

## Alternative Names

*Calcis. Calc.*
Calcium ion ($Ca^{2+}$).
Lime.
Electrolyte.
Mineral.

## Nature

Calcium is classified as an alkaline earth metal in the s-block, group 2 (IIA), period 4, of the periodic table of elements. It exists as a divalent cation $Ca^{2+}$. This is the only form of interest as far nutrition is concerned, although it may exist either as the free ion (in trace amounts and contribute slightly to the electrolyte content of biological fluids) or it may be bound to various molecules, including citrate and proteins. Magnesium Mg, is another member of the group.

## Biological Functions

- Calcium is the most abundant mineral in the human body.

- Ninety percent of the calcium in the body is found in the bones and teeth. It is perhaps of interest here to describe the composition of bone in some detail. Human bone consists of about 45 percent water, 25 percent inorganic material, 20 percent protein and 10 percent lipid. The inorganic material may be extracted by ashing the bone. In terms of simple chemicals this ash may be considered to consist of 84 percent calcium phosphate; 10 percent calcium carbonate; 2 percent calcium citrate; 2 percent sodium phosphate; 1 percent magnesium phosphate and 1 percent magnesium carbonate. Bone is a complex crystal of these elements called hydroxyapatite, which may in addition contain minute traces of other elements particularly fluoride. Strictly pure hydroxyapatite contains only 40 percent calcium; 57 percent phosphate and 3 percent hydroxide. It should be noted that only one third of the phosphate is elemental phosphorous the form in which it is specified in dietary tables. When this is taken into account, it can be seen that calcium is the predominant mineral in bone. Therefore, the exact ratio of elemental calcium to elemental phosphorous in bone is nearer 2 to 1.

- Calcium is essential for muscle contraction and nerve transmission. The concentration of calcium (and magnesium) across the cell membrane determines the excitability of muscle and nerve cells, particularly at their junctions. In this context, excessive calcium causes rigor whereas lack of calcium causes tetany.

- Calcium is essential for blood clotting. It acts on blood platelets to release thromboplastin which is the first enzyme in a series culminating in the formation of the clot matrix called fibrin after blood is shed. If calcium is removed from the blood it will not clot. The Blood Bank exploits this effect to good advantage when storing blood for transfusions.

- Calcium helps the body to utilize iron. It helps the absorption of vitamin $B_{12}$ which is essential in this process.

- The level of calcium in the blood is controlled by both vitamin D and the hormone secreted by the parathyroid gland called the parathyroid hormone.

- Calcium helps maintain the integrity of cell membranes and cytoplasmic substances by combining with the phospholipid, lecithin. In this way, it controls the permeability of the cell to various nutrients.

- Calcium is involved in the activation or inhibition of many enzymes. In this role, it often works with magnesium. It also appears to function on its own. For example, it activates the digestive enzyme called lipase which breaks down neutral fats (triglycerides) in the small intestine. Like magnesium it also activates some enzymes which are involved in carbohydrate metabolism.

- An intracellular protein called calmodulin which is widely distributed in both animals and plants has been found to play a key role in the activation of enzymes by calcium. Calcium ions bind to calmodulin in a 4 to 1 ratio and the complex then binds to various enzymes to regulate their activity. The enzymes involved include the muscle enzyme myosin light-chain kinase, calcium activated ATPase, NAD kinase, microtubule disassembly enzyme, membrane phosphorylation enzyme, calcium dependent protein kinase, and many others. The role of calmodulin in activating microtubule disassembly is believed to involve aiding the chromosomes to separate during cell division. Its role in activating myosin kinase is essential for smooth muscle contraction. Interestingly, calmodulin does not occur in skeletal or heart muscle but another protein called troponin C is involved and this protein is structurally related to calmodulin. Calmodulin has a unique feature in that one of its amino acid components is a trimethylated lysine residue. This involves a post-translational modification in the lysine residue.

- Calcium and, indeed, phosphate metabolism cannot be adequately considered without reference to vitamin D and a number of hormones most particularly the parathyroid hormone and calcitonin. These aspects are dealt with in detail later in Part 3, Chapter 60.

## Requirement

The turnover of calcium in bone is of the order of 700 mg per day in typical adults, but the amount of calcium lost from the body is generally much less than this. Individual requirements of this nutrient vary considerably. Values from 200 to 1,000 milligrams per day may be required to maintain calcium balance. The recommended adult daily intake of calcium in both males and in females is 1.0 g/d. High dietary intake of phosphorous or protein may increase calcium loss. Children require up to four times more calcium per kilogram of body weight than adults. Marked increases in calcium are also required for pregnancy or lactation in women. It is often considered that older people should take additional calcium, although there is some disagreement on this point. As a rule, every gram of calcium should be accompanied by one gram of phosphorous in the diet for adults. Whereas for young infants the ratio should be nearer 3 grams of calcium for every 2 grams of phosphorous, as is provided in human milk. The major food source of calcium is milk and its products, especially cheese. In general, over 80 percent of the daily calcium requirement is derived from this source.

Both calcium and magnesium are lost during the refining of foodstuffs. Also, calcium and magnesium absorption is reduced in the presence of phytin. Phytin is a phosphate derivative of inositol. Usually six phosphate residues combine with the inositol. Phytate is the mixed calcium and magnesium salt of phytin. In many animals, a digestive enzyme called phytase is required to break down this salt before absorption of its components can take place. Ruminants such as cattle and sheep have the greatest activity of the enzyme phytase, but most animals including humans have some phytase activity. The enzyme also occurs in several cereal grains and may break down phytin during certain cooking processes. Hence there is less concern for the presence of phytin in foods than in the past.

Calcium absorption from the gut may be enhanced by the presence of the milk sugar lactose. This is of relevance particularly in young children. The ratio of calcium to phosphorous in the diet also influences their respective rates of absorption. Too much of either calcium or phosphorous tends to inhibit absorption by forming insoluble calcium phosphate salts in the gut. However, ratios anywhere in the range from about 2:1 down to about 1:2 do not appear to have any adverse effect, and even more extreme ratios can be tolerated provided sufficient vitamin D is contained in the diet. In the typical Western diet, the ratio of calcium to phosphorous lies generally between about 1:1.2 on the one hand and 1:1.9 on the other. In fact, the most ideal ratio is not yet known for human nutrition. Some authors have hinted that a slightly higher level of calcium would be beneficial for prolonged intakes. About 60 percent of our daily requirement of calcium comes from milk and cheese, a further 23 percent comes from grain and its products notably bread. A calcium compendium is included for reference (Table 33.1). Calcium is lost by excretion mainly in the faeces, but a small amount is lost in the urine and in the sweat, particularly in hot climates.

## Toxicity

A toxicity of calcium is termed hypercalcemia. This is relatively rare in normal individuals where it probably never occurs. A toxicity of calcium can occur indirectly as a complication of vitamin D toxicity (see Chapter 60). Diseases of the parathyroid glands leading to excessive secretion of the parathyroid hormone may also cause calcium toxicity to occur. Also, certain types of cancer cells appear to be able to produce the parathyroid hormone with similar results. Excessive intake of calcium, say over 2 grams per day for extended periods, may produce some toxic symptoms. High levels of calcium in the blood tend to depress the levels of phosphate. Also, calcium toxicity may result in a deposition of calcium in the soft tissues including the heart, aorta and kidneys. Excessive calcium may inhibit the absorption of other minerals.

## Deficiency

A deficiency of calcium is termed hypocalcemia. Excessive intake of foods containing phosphates, oxalate and possibly phytates, tend to form insoluble salts of calcium and magnesium that decrease their rate of absorption. Although there is some evidence that the human body can adapt to a regular intake of phytin-containing foods. Protein tends to assist calcium absorption but very high protein intakes also increase the urinary loss of calcium. Excessive intakes of fat or inadequate fat absorption may interfere with calcium absorption. Excessive intake of magnesium results in an increased loss of calcium in the urine, and *vice versa*.

Daily intakes of calcium as low as 400 milligrams over extended periods do not appear to produce a deficiency in many humans. Part of the explanation lies in the fact that most adults appear to be able to adapt to low intakes of calcium. One reason could be the fact that relatively more calcium is absorbed from a poor diet than from a rich one.

In young children lack of calcium or phosphorous or insufficient vitamin D can result in rickets, the most noticeable symptom of which is bowed legs. In adults, any of these deficiencies result in osteomalacia which is a similar condition but without the bending of bones (which are already formed). There is in fact little loss of bone mass but the structure of the bone is altered and it tends to fracture easily. Older women can suffer from a calcium and phosphorous loss from bone called osteoporosis which also results in brittle bones as well as a generalized decrease in bone mass. The consequences of a lack of calcium parallel those of a lack of phosphate regarding bone metabolism.

A lack of exercise causes a loss of calcium from the bones even in persons on an adequate calcium diet. Loss of bone mineralization in the jaw, leading to periodontal disease and tooth decay or loss may occur in extreme cases. Immobilisation is one form of lack of exercise that may affect one limb for example after a breakage. Bed rest is another that affects the whole body. People who lead sedentary lives and stay indoors a lot may also not be getting enough exercise to maintain calcium balance.

High phosphate intakes tend to result in large losses of calcium in the faeces. Vitamin D is essential for the adequate absorption and retention of calcium. A deficiency of calcium has the same effect on bone as a deficiency of phosphate or vitamin D. These effects are considered in the following chapter. A deficiency of calcium may cause insomnia in certain individuals and pains in the muscles and joints. In young children, there may be sweating and lethargy. In adults, other more general symptoms include depression and anxiety.

A deficiency of calcium in the blood results in nerve and muscle disorders including tetany which can lead to death if not corrected. In this regard, the effects of a lack of calcium and magnesium are very similar and are difficult to distinguish from each other.

**Table 33.1.** Calcium compendium

| FOOD GROUP | CALCIUM LEVEL |
|---|---|
| Milk / Products | Medium / Very high |
| Eggs | Low |
| Meat and fish | Very low |
| Fats and oils | Nil |
| Grain / Products | Low / Medium |
| Nuts / Pulses | High / Medium |
| Root vegetables | Low |
| Leaf vegetables | Medium, variable |
| Fruit | Very low |
| Sweets | Nil |

# 34

# PHOSPHOROUS

## Common Name

Phosphorous (elemental), (P).

## Alternative Names

Orthophosphate, $P_i$ ("$PO_4$").
Inorganic Phosphorous / Phosphate. Phosphoric (acid).
*Phos.*
Mineral. Electrolyte.

## Nature

Phosphorous is classified as a nonmetal in the p-block, group 15 (VB), period 3, of the periodic table of elements. It is in the same group as nitrogen N and arsenic As. The predominant form of phosphorous is the orthophosphate anion which occurs either as the monovalent anion $H_2PO_4^-$, or the divalent anion $HPO_4^{2-}$. These are interconvertible depending on the acidity, and allow phosphate to contribute to the electrolyte content of many biological fluids. For example, in blood plasma at pH 7.4, there is approximately four times more of the divalent form relative to the monovalent form. Together, they are referred to as inorganic phosphorous, orthophosphate, or simply phosphate $P_i$. This is the form of interest as far as mineral nutrition is concerned. Organic forms of phosphate also occur but these are not considered as being independently essential, because they can all be synthesised in the body from inorganic phosphorous. Sometimes, there is confusion regarding the exact form in which phosphorous is measured. The term phosphate is often used to mean

34

the inorganic phosphorous. Strictly speaking, daily intakes and so on, refer to the total amount of phosphorous occurring in all forms. Most of the inorganic form is orthophosphate. While organic forms yield inorganic forms in the digestive tract and subsequently these can also be absorbed.

## Biological Functions

* Phosphorous has more functions than any other mineral in the body.

* Inorganic phosphorous occurs predominantly as the phosphate ion. Phosphorous as phosphate is the second most abundant mineral in the human body. Phosphorous in this form is very closely linked with calcium metabolism. Approximately 20 percent of the body phosphorous occurs as phosphate, and of this, 85 percent is found in bone. Further details on bone are given in the following chapter on calcium. Phosphorous also occurs in a multitude of less tangible organic forms where it is essential for almost all life processes.

* Phosphorous occurs in the genetic material nucleic acid, which is essential for cell growth and the elaboration of all cellular proteins including enzymes.

* Phosphorous can form high energy bonds within molecules. In this form, it plays a crucial role in storing energy for synthetic reactions involved in growth and metabolism. The key high energy coinage of the living cell is called adenosine triphosphate (ATP), which is an organic molecule containing three units of phosphate linked in sequence. A secondary store of energy in the body is creatine phosphate. Creatine phosphate increases the capacity of the body to store readily available energy in muscle cells by a factor of some seven times.

* Like chloride, inorganic phosphate is negatively charged carrying one or two negative charges depending on the acidity of the environment. Phosphate contributes significantly to the electrolyte content of the cell.

* Phosphorous is intimately involved in carbohydrate metabolism. It acts by combining with carbohydrate units to form

35

metabolically active phosphates.

- Phosphate is an integral component of several phospholipids such as lecithin.

- Phosphate is associated with several proteins, in particular the milk protein casein, where it is found together with calcium.

- The phosphate anion can exist in two forms under physiological conditions namely dihydrogen phosphate, $H_2PO_4^-$ and hydrogen phosphate $HPO_4^{2-}$ , respectively. These forms are interconvertible by the combination or removal of a single hydrogen ion $H^+$. Therefore, phosphates play a key role in regulating acid-base balance in the body, and in eliminating excess acid in the urine.

- Although phosphorous does not activate or inhibit enzymes in the control sense, it is often found as an integral component of them. It functions as part of certain enzymes and is therefore essential to the activity of these enzymes.

- The level of phosphate in the blood is influenced by both vitamin D and the parathyroid hormone.

## Requirement

There is a strong metabolic link between phosphorous and calcium. In fact, the average daily intake of phosphorous in the Western diet probably exceeds the calcium intake. Typical phosphorous intakes range from about 800 to 1,500 milligrams per day in adults. Only in young infants are relatively lower values of phosphorous than calcium recommended, as found in human milk. The recommended adult daily intake of phosphorous in both males and in females is 700 mg/d.

Phosphorous is universally distributed in food. A phosphorous compendium is included for reference (Table 34.1). About 10 percent of the total dietary phosphate in Western diets comes from added phosphates in processed foods. Up to 90 percent of the phosphate released by the digestion of food may be absorbed.

## Toxicity

A toxicity of phosphorous is termed hyperphosphatemia. Phosphate toxicity is rare in normal individuals but can occur as a complication of kidney failure. The symptoms include a disturbance of the calcium to phosphate ratio in the blood tending to decrease the levels of calcium. This is caused by a reduction in the level of a vitamin D metabolite called 1, 25-dihydroxyvitamin $D_3$ as will be considered in Chapter 60. Acute phosphate toxicity can result in hypocalcaemia and associated symptoms including tetany, high blood pressure and increased heart rate. Prolonged moderate phosphate toxicity can lead to a usually irreversible deposition of calcium phosphate crystals in various soft tissues including the heart. Excessive intakes of phosphorous can inhibit the absorption of other minerals notably calcium, zinc and iron.

## Deficiency

A phosphorous deficiency is termed hypophosphatemia. In fact, a deficiency of phosphorous is virtually unknown in normal individuals, even though pregnancy and lactation can add extra demands for phosphate in the diet. However, excessive use of antacids for indigestion may make phosphorous in food less available for absorption. This is because antacids combine with phosphate to form insoluble salts. In cattle, a phosphorous deficiency occasionally occurs and one of the first symptoms is that the animals chew at rocks, wood and even bones. During chronic deficiency of phosphorous there is a gradual weakening of bones which become painful causing stiffness and lameness.

In young children lack of calcium or phosphorous or insufficient vitamin D can result in rickets, the most noticeable symptom of which is bowed legs. In adults, any of these deficiencies result in osteomalacia which is a similar condition but without the bending of bones (which are already formed). There is in fact little loss of bone mass but the structure of the bone is altered and it tends to fracture easily. Older women can suffer from a calcium and phosphorous loss from bone called osteoporosis which also results in brittle bones as well as a generalized decrease in bone mass. The consequences of a lack of phosphorous therefore parallel those of a lack of calcium regarding bone metabolism. Additional calcium with vitamin D can prove beneficial in some of these cases. Supplements containing up to one gram of calcium per day are often recommended.

**Table 34.1.** Phosphorous compendium

| FOOD GROUP | PHOSPHOROUS LEVEL |
| --- | --- |
| Milk / Products | Low / Very high |
| Eggs | Medium |
| Meat and fish | Medium |
| Fats and oils | Nil |
| Grain and products | Medium |
| Nuts and pulses | Very high |
| Root vegetables | Low |
| Leaf vegetables | Low |
| Fruit | Very low |
| Sweets | Nil |

# 35

# MAGNESIUM

## Common Name

Magnesium (elemental), (Mg).

## Alternative Names

*Magnesia. Mag.*
Magnesium ion ($Mg^{2+}$).
Electrolyte.
Mineral.

## Nature

Magnesium is classified as an alkaline earth metal in the s-block, group 2 (IIA), period 3, of the periodic table of elements. It exists as the divalent cation $Mg^{2+}$. This is the only form of interest as far as nutrition is concerned. Magnesium is in the same group as calcium Ca, and may contribute slightly to the electrolyte content of some fluids.

## Biological Functions

- Magnesium is the second most abundant intracellular cation after potassium.

- Magnesium activates or inhibits several enzymes and is essential for the activity of other enzymes. Altogether, magnesium is involved in over 300 enzyme reactions. Enzymes called kinases and phosphatases involved in the reactions of phosphate groups require magnesium. Magnesium activates deoxyribonuclease but

40

it inhibits ribonuclease. These enzymes are essential in nucleic acid metabolism. Magnesium is an essential component of arginase, the enzyme which converts the amino acid arginine to urea. Highly specific phosphate enzymes called ATPases may either be activated by magnesium and inhibited by calcium or *vice versa* depending on their location in the cell. Magnesium is also required for several enzymes involved in carbohydrate metabolism.

- Magnesium is a key electrolyte in the sense that it maintains the excitability of cell membranes particularly those of nerve and muscle. As a general rule, decreasing the calcium or magnesium level outside the nerve cell causes an increase in the excitability of the membrane. However, calcium ions promote the release of nerve transmitters at the nerve endings whereas magnesium ions tend to oppose this release.

- Magnesium regulates normal heart rhythm and has been used to treat arrhythmia (irregular heartbeat).

- Magnesium and calcium are closely related chemically, both being divalent cations of the Group IIA elements. They share several mechanisms of transport and excretion in the body.

- Up to 60 percent of the magnesium in the body is found in bone.

- Magnesium and calcium work together to reduce irritability by helping the enzyme choline esterase break down excessive amounts of acetylcholine, which is the nerve transmitter at cholinergic or parasympathetic nerve endings.

- Magnesium appears to alleviate premenstrual symptoms.

- There is evidence that magnesium supplementation can improve insulin sensitivity in diabetics and help regulate blood sugar levels.

## Requirement

The intake of magnesium in a typical Western diet varies from about 25 to 35 milligrams per 1,000 kilojoules (or 110 to 140 milligrams per 1,000 kilocalories). At this level of intake, there is no risk of magnesium deficiency. For adults, approximately 30 milligrams of magnesium per 1,000 kJ is recommended. Estimates of adult dietary needs under different conditions can vary from as little as 200 mg per day to as much as 700 mg per day. It seems that the average requirement is about 5 mg per day per kg of body weight. On average, a ratio of about 2 mg of magnesium to every 5 mg of calcium is adequate to maintain balance in adults. The recommended adult daily intake of magnesium in males is 420 mg/d and in females is 320 mg/d, respectively. Increased intake of magnesium is required during pregnancy and lactation. The values recommended are based on corresponding calcium intakes. However, it may be assumed that if the correct calcium intakes are provided then magnesium levels should also be adequate. Magnesium is absorbed from the small intestine and may be excreted in the faeces and to a lesser extent in the urine.

For a wide range of foods, the levels of magnesium and calcium are comparable. Vegetables are a rich source of magnesium. A magnesium compendium is included for reference (Table 35.1). However, magnesium never reaches the highest levels found for calcium in certain foods. Like calcium, magnesium is lost during the refining of foods.

## Toxicity

A toxicity of magnesium is termed hypermagnesemia. Magnesium is relatively non-toxic. Large doses in the range 3 to 5 grams of magnesium salts may result in diarrhoea (which had been used as a therapeutic effect for constipation). Excessive intake of magnesium may promote the excretion of calcium. A toxicity of magnesium may develop as a result of kidney failure. Intakes of 3 grams per day may cause toxicity in these patients. The principle symptom is a generalized depression of the nervous system including shallow breathing and ultimately death.

## Deficiency

A deficiency of magnesium is termed hypomagnesemia, but is rare in humans. A deficiency can result as a complication of kwashiorkor (protein-energy malnutrition), or chronic diarrhoea of any origin. Similarly, alcoholics often exhibit a magnesium deficiency, particularly if they do not eat properly. Some women on the contraceptive pill have been found to have a deficiency of magnesium. Lack of magnesium particularly in infants may result in tremor and even convulsions. Magnesium deficiency may also result in behavioural modifications. A number of drugs can affect the magnesium level in the body. Excessive intake of calcium results in an increased loss of magnesium in the urine, and *vice versa*.

Deficiency of magnesium results in many symptoms including generalised weakness, nervousness, cramps in the muscles, loss of balance, palpitations and low blood sugar. A lack of magnesium has been found in the heart muscle of certain heart attack victims. However, the significance of this finding is still uncertain. Migraine sufferers also tend to have lower magnesium levels. Magnesium deficiency is known to inhibit vitamin D metabolism and cause calcium depletion. Magnesium deficiency is linked to low blood levels of potassium. Deficiency symptoms of magnesium tend to progress as follows. There may be a drop in blood pressure due to vasodilation often accompanied by a flushed appearance of the skin. Then a generalised hyperirritability may develop leading finally to tetany and death. In calves, a similar magnesium tetany called 'grass staggers' may result from a joint magnesium and calcium deficiency.

**Table 35.1.** Magnesium compendium

| FOOD GROUP | MAGNESIUM LEVEL |
| --- | --- |
| Milk and products | Low |
| Eggs | Very low |
| Meat and fish | Low |
| Fats and oils | Nil |
| Grain and products | High |
| Nuts and pulses | Very high |
| Root vegetables | Low |
| Leaf vegetables | Low |
| Fruit | Very low |
| Sweets | Nil |

# 36

# IRON

## Common Name

Iron (elemental), (Fe).

## Alternative Names

*Ferrum, Fer.*
Ferrous ion ($Fe^{2+}$). Ferric ion ($Fe^{3+}$).
Mineral.
Trace element.

## Nature

Iron is classified as a transition metal in the d-block, group 8 (VIII), period 4, of the periodic table of elements. It is a transition element of the first series. It occurs in two main cationic forms, ferrous $Fe^{2+}$, and ferric $Fe^{3+}$, which are readily interconvertible. These arise from the oxidation states Fe(II) and Fe(III), respectively. The symbol for iron comes from the Latin word *ferrum*.

## Biological Functions

- Iron was the very first mineral to be recognised as essential in humans. In 1831, it was realised that a lack of iron could cause anaemia.

- Iron occurs in two reversible ionic forms, ferrous and ferric. Per kilogram of body weight, about 35 milligrams of iron occur in haemoglobin, myoglobin and enzymes. About half this amount again occurs in ferritin and hemosiderin which are the main stores of iron in the body. Put another way, about 65 percent of the iron in the body is found in haemoglobin, 10 percent in myoglobin, 10 percent in ferritin, 9 percent in hemosiderin, 5 percent in miscellaneous substances and 1 percent in enzymes and electron carrier proteins.

- As stated above, iron is a constituent of the oxygen carrying protein called haemoglobin which gives blood its red colour. This is by far the best-known function of iron; it's role in the supply of oxygen to cells and muscles in the body. Haemoglobin is composed of 96 percent protein (globin) and 4 percent haem (complexed iron).

- Iron is also a component of myoglobin the oxygen carrying protein found in muscles.

- Several enzymes contain iron which is essential for their function. These include various peroxidases which break down toxic peroxides in the body, xanthine oxidase which also contains molybdenum and produces uric acid from the purines, and certain dehydrogenases involved in carbohydrate metabolism.

- Iron is an essential cofactor in the production of neurotransmitters like noradrenaline, serotonin, and dopamine.

- Some electron transfer proteins also contain iron. The main iron containing electron carriers are called cytochromes and are found in the mitochondria. Essential to their function is the reversible ferrous/ferric reaction which enables the high energy of free electrons released during metabolism to be harnessed to produce ATP. These carriers also transfer the accompanying free hydrogens (protons) released during metabolism to oxygen to form water in the cell. This water is termed metabolic water, as considered in Part 1, Chapters 4 and 7.

- Iron is required for the optimum functioning of the immune system, and resistance to disease and infections.

## Requirement

In adults, the daily loss of iron is limited to about 1 mg per day in skin and intestinal cells. Because of this limited rate of loss from the body, the main way in which iron levels are controlled in the body is through the regulation of iron absorption. Normally, very little iron, amounting to less than 10 percent in the diet, is absorbed. Although, in certain circumstances, the rate of absorption can be increased by 2 to 3 times during periods of deficiency, but even this is not always sufficient to prevent anaemia from occurring.

The average uptake of iron varies from about 1 - 2 mg per 1,000 kJ (or 5 - 8 mg per 1,000 kcal) of food intake. Men absorb only 5 to 7 percent of the total iron in their diet, whereas women may absorb up to 13 percent. Total body stores of iron average about 1,000 mg in men and 300 mg in women. A body store of 300 mg iron would be sufficient to sustain an individual for several months on a very low dietary intake. The recommended adult daily intake of iron in males is 8 mg/d and in females is 18 mg/d, respectively. These amounts meet most nutritional requirements of healthy adults. In women, iron is required to replace menstrual blood loss. Pregnant women need extra iron, which is utilised by the growing baby. Lactation does not require additional amounts of iron because even though the volume of milk (up to 800 ml per day), is high the concentration of iron in the milk is very low and the total loss in milk is less than the menstrual blood loss.

Iron may be absorbed either combined as haem (a component of haemoglobin and myoglobin) or as free inorganic iron. About 40% of the total iron in animal tissues is in the haem form and the remainder occurs as non-haem compounds, whereas all the iron in plants is in the non-haem form. Haem and non-haem iron are absorbed by different mechanisms. The haem form is highly absorbable and the inorganic ferrous form is more readily absorbed than the ferric form.

After absorption of the ferrous form mainly in the duodenum and upper small intestine, it is oxidised to the ferric form which is bound to various carrier proteins. The three principle carriers are the mucosal protein (intracellular carrier), the iron storage protein (ferritin) and the blood plasma carrier protein (transferrin). The mucosal carrier can take up more iron during iron deficiencies but has a maximum capacity during iron overload. Therefore, it functions as a protective natural barrier to excess iron uptake from the diet. A second carrier protein, apoferritin, can combine with over 4,000 iron atoms to form ferritin, which is the principle store of iron in the body. Another carrier called apotransferrin binds just 2 iron atoms to form transferrin, but this is the principle carrier of iron in the blood plasma. It is the transferrin which carries iron to the bone marrow, spleen or liver storage sites where ferritin is found.

Generally, the various stores of iron in the body are in equilibrium with each other and iron can be recycled in the body. But some iron is lost mainly in the faeces and traces are also excreted in the urine and in sweat. In fact, the loss of iron per day varies from person to person. It has been estimated that the average daily turnover of iron is 14 µg/kg body weight in men and 22 µg/kg body weight in women. Adult men lose from 0.4 to 2.0 mg per day with an average value around 1 mg per day. On average, adult women lose an additional 0.5 mg per day (because of menstruation). In other words, an intake of 0.5 mg per day for a full month is required to replace the amount lost during each menstrual cycle on average. Some women lose less than this but a small percentage of women can lose up to three times this amount per month but the recommended intake of 18 mg/day should provide sufficient iron for almost all women. Nevertheless, a small number of women (not more than 5%) with exceptionally high menstrual losses may require an additional intake, possibly in the form of iron supplements. Assuming 10 percent absorption for example, 30 - 60 mg iron as a supplement should provide some 3 - 6 mg additional iron per day. Pregnancy increases the daily requirement of iron to some 2 to 4 mg (average 3.5 mg). Lactation requires an additional 0.15 to 0.3 mg per day which is less than the value required during menstruation. Up to 2 mg additional iron per day is required for rapidly growing male children. And, an additional 5 mg per day is required for rapidly growing female children.

About 40 percent of our iron requirement comes from grain and its products. Another 24 percent comes from meat, particularly red meat, and about 18 percent comes from vegetables particularly greens. An iron compendium is included for reference (Table 36.1).

## Toxicity

48

Iron toxicity is rare in humans. Average intakes of iron in the diet in the range 10 to 25 mg per day do not produce any toxic effects in adults. Iron is toxic, particularly in young children, if intake is excessive. One effect of excess iron is the conversion of ferritin to hemosiderin. In cases of excessive uptake some of the ferritin is denatured and precipitated to form giant particles called hemosiderin which are less efficient at iron exchange than ferritin. Hemosiderin may appear in the liver, pancreas and even in the skin and joints. Excessive formation of hemosiderin is called hemosiderosis.

A rare genetic disorder of iron absorption where the natural mucosal barrier is affected also leads to iron intoxication over many years. Excessive deposits of hemosiderin form throughout the body which eventually disrupt normal function and can cause significant organ damage. This condition is called hemochromatosis.

## Deficiency

Milk has a low iron content and prolonged breast-feeding may result in iron deficiency in infants over the age of six months. Iron deficiency is the most common mineral deficiency in adults particularly women throughout the world. A deficiency of iron may be caused indirectly by the lack of adequate amounts of certain vitamins such as folate and vitamin $B_{12}$. The lack of reducing substances in the diet, such as vitamin C, decrease the conversion of ferric to ferrous iron, and consequently decrease the rate of absorption of iron in general. A lack of iron may predispose to lowered resistance to infection. Iron deficiency in women is mostly caused by the low rate of absorption of iron rather than the lack of iron in the diet. Anaemia is caused by a chronic iron deficiency. However, there are several types of anaemia which must be clinically distinguished from each other. Iron deficiency anaemia is one of the common forms of nutritional anaemias. Further comments on anaemias are included in the chapter on links between the vitamins and the minerals (Part 3, Chapter 62).

**Table 36.1.** Iron compendium

| FOOD GROUP | IRON LEVEL |
| --- | --- |
| Milk and products | Very low |
| Eggs | Medium |
| Meat /<br>Fish | Very high, variable /<br>Low, variable |
| Fats and oils | Nil |
| Grain and products | Medium, variable |
| Nuts and pulses | Very high |
| Root vegetables | Low |
| Leaf vegetables | Medium, variable |
| Fruit | Very low |
| Sweets | Very low, variable |

Iron values are very variable.

# 37

# ZINC

## Common Name

Zinc (elemental), (Zn).

## Alternative Names

Zinc ion ($Zn^{2+}$).
Mineral.
Trace element.

## Nature

Zinc is classified as a metal in the d-block, group 12 (IIB), period 4, of the periodic table of elements. It occurs as a divalent cation $Zn^{2+}$. This is the only form of interest in nutrition. Cadmium Cd, is another member of the group.

## Biological Functions

*   Zinc was first recognised as essential to plants in 1869. It was sometime later that it was realised to be essential in humans. In 1940, Keilin and Mann showed that zinc was an essential component of the carbonic anhydrase enzyme. Zinc came into its own in the 1950's when it was discovered that a lack of zinc caused nanism (a form of dwarfism) in humans.

*   Zinc is involved in the action of over a hundred enzymes involved in all areas of metabolism. Some of these include alcohol-, lactate- and glutamate dehydrogenases, alkaline phosphatase, superoxide dismutase, pancreatic carboxypeptidase, thymidine kinase and carbonic anhydrase. Superoxide dismutase

is an important antioxidant enzyme which protects the body against the harmful effects of free radicals. Free radicals are short-lived but very active fragments of molecules containing a charge and which usually contain oxygen. These fragments cause a loss of membrane integrity in various cells and organelles.

- Zinc is essential to the formation of certain prostaglandins. It has been suggested that the lack of zinc-induced prostaglandin formation may result in acne which is a common scourge during the adolescent years. Zinc is involved in certain processes of the immune system, hence its claim to be of help in reducing the incidence or symptoms of the common cold. Certain prostaglandins (the Series-I type) act as mediators in this effect. Zinc also helps to maintain the balance of activity of the different types of prostaglandins. The first step where zinc acts in this process is the conversion of the precursor linoleic acid to gamma-linoleic acid (see also Part 1, Chapter 15, on the essential fatty acids).

- Another possible role for zinc in ameliorating the effects of the common cold may be its ability to inhibit the release of histamine. Histamine is a natural irritant which is released from certain cells following injury or infection. This may also explain the role of zinc in relieving certain forms of allergy. Although the mechanism of action of zinc in this regard is not yet fully understood.

- Zinc has a role to play in the specialisation of the lymphocytes; the white cells that fight infection. It is believed that zinc is essential for the action of certain thymus gland hormones which are involved in this process. Several cases have been reported where zinc supplements have boosted the immune system in both infants and adults. Zinc is also essential for the healing of wounds.

- Zinc is involved in nucleic acid and protein metabolism. Collagen is one of the essential structural proteins that zinc helps to synthesise. Collagen is found in bone and in connective tissue. Zinc is also essential for aspects of lipid and carbohydrate metabolism.

- Zinc is required for the efficient release of insulin, the sugar controlling hormone, from the pancreas. Zinc is also involved in the metabolism of several hormones of the pituitary gland and the reproductive glands. In the latter, zinc is essential to produce sperm in the testes and the maturation of ova in the ovaries. Therefore, zinc is essential for various aspects of human sexual development and reproduction in both the male and the female. Regarding female physiology, zinc is involved in areas of menstruation, foetal growth during pregnancy and lactation.

- Zinc helps to mobilise vitamin A which is stored in the liver, and therefore helps to maintain night vision.

- Zinc may serve as an antioxidant through its relationship to superoxide dismutase. Apart from zinc, selenium also works as an antioxidant. Two vitamins namely, vitamin C and vitamin E, also serve a major role in protecting the body from free radicals. The long-term effects of even small traces of free radicals may include atherosclerosis and cancer.

- Zinc may protect the body against the harmful effects of certain heavy metals such as cadmium, lead and mercury which are highly toxic.

- Zinc may help relieve the symptoms of depression in certain individuals, and may also help with other mental disorders possibly even schizophrenia.

- Zinc has been used recently in the treatment of herpes. It has been found that zinc inhibits the replication of the herpes simplex (cold sore) virus.

- Zinc is necessary for the development of nervous tissue including the brain itself.

- Zinc is required for the proper functioning of our sense of taste and smell. Recently a zinc deficiency test based on the ability to detect a dilute chemical solution has been developed. Just 1 gram of zinc sulphate dissolved in 1 litre of distilled water should have a distinctive taste which some people find unpleasant. People who are zinc deficient will either taste nothing or take several seconds before perceiving the taste. Such persons could benefit from zinc supplementation. People who immediately detect the taste are not zinc deficient.

## Requirement

Studies show that the bioavailability of zinc varies considerably. A zinc compendium is included for reference (Table 37.1). It is assumed that on average about 40 percent of the zinc in the diet is absorbed. There is an increased requirement for zinc during pregnancy and lactation. Also, extra zinc may be needed during illness and old age. The typical Western diet does not always contain sufficient zinc to supply these needs. The recommended adult daily intake of zinc in males is 11 mg/d and in females is 8 mg/d, respectively.

Phytin reduces the rate of absorption of zinc as it does calcium. There is a high content of phytin in bran for example. It has been suggested that zinc may bind to a factor secreted by the pancreas which promotes zinc absorption. Like iron, zinc can be stored in the mucosal cells by zinc carrier proteins. Zinc is secreted into the gut by pancreatic juice and is thus eliminated in the faeces. It has been claimed that picolinic acid, a derivative of the amino acid tryptophan, dramatically increases the ability to absorb zinc from the gut.

A greater intake of zinc is required if the intake of essential fatty acids is inadequate. More zinc may be required if the diet is low in certain vitamins especially vitamin C and vitamin $B_6$. Excessive calcium or phosphate intake may also reduce zinc absorption. About 43 percent of our zinc requirement is obtained from meat, and a further 29 percent comes from milk and cheese products, about 15 percent derives from grain products and a further 8 percent from various vegetables.

## Toxicity

Toxicity due to zinc is relatively rare in humans. Although intakes in the range 10 to 25 mg per day are common and in the recommended range, it is not recommended to take over 150 mg regularly per day because of the risk of other mineral imbalances that this could create. In this regard, copper deficiency could be the most serious effect. Excessive zinc may also suppress iron absorption. possible Peripheral neuropathy, with loss of sensation in extremities may occur in extreme cases.

## Deficiency

The symptoms of zinc deficiency include a general apathy, learning difficulties, a dulling of the sense of taste and sometimes the sense of smell leading to poor appetite. Other symptoms include poor healing of wounds, anaemia, the appearance of white spots or bands on the nails which become brittle, night blindness, general jitteriness and an increased susceptibility to infections. There may be an elevated ribonuclease enzyme activity but reduced red blood cell carbonic anhydrase enzyme activity.

Zinc is essential to the growth of infants and even a lack of zinc in the mother during pregnancy can lead to abnormalities in the growing foetus. Some individuals have a reduced ability to absorb zinc and may thus tend to become deficient. Zinc deficiency may result in stunted growth leading to a form of dwarfism called nanism, poor hair growth, coarsening of the skin and a lack of sexual development.

A very rare inherited condition called acrodermatitis entropathica apparently causes food proteins, except those found in human milk, to bind with zinc. Bottle fed infants with this disease develop persistent diarrhoea and wounds on the skin. This can be offset by feeding supplements of zinc to overcome the binding effect. It has been discovered that the amino acid L-histidine combines with zinc and has the therapeutic effect of reducing appetite which may help certain people to lose weight but this should only be carried out under strict supervision because of the risk of becoming zinc deficient.

Zinc deficiency is more frequent in people with the genetic disorders of sickle cell anaemia and Downs syndrome. Strict vegetarians (vegans) also run the risk of becoming zinc deficient. Diabetic patients have been found to have less zinc the normal individuals. Alcoholics have also been found to have lower zinc levels, because alcohol interferes with zinc absorption and increases the rate of zinc loss from the body. The contraceptive pill tends to cause a zinc deficiency in the blood plasma. Excessive copper in drinking water can prevent zinc absorption and thus lead to a deficiency. Milking mothers, in the first few weeks after birth, require extra zinc. Following the extra requirements during pregnancy, milking may thus result in deficiency in some cases. Low zinc levels are common in patients with anorexia nervosa. But the interpretation of this observation is uncertain at present. It could be caused by the general lack of food over time rather than be the direct cause of the condition. In another study, it was found that zinc deficiency may be a factor contributing to some forms of high blood pressure.

**Table 37.1.** Zinc compendium

| FOOD GROUP | ZINC LEVEL |
| --- | --- |
| Milk / Products | Very low / Very variable |
| Eggs | Medium |
| Meat and fish | Very variable |
| Fats and oils | Nil |
| Grain and products | High, variable |
| Nuts and pulses | High |
| Root vegetables | Low |
| Leaf vegetables | Low, variable |
| Fruit | Very low |
| Sweets | Nil |

Zinc levels are very variable.

# 38

# FLUORIDE

## Common Name

Fluoride (ion), (F$^-$).

## Alternative Names

Elemental (not gaseous) fluorine (F, not F$_2$).
Mineral.
Trace Element.

## Nature

Fluorine is classified as a nonmetal in the p-block, group VIIB, period 2, of the periodic table of elements. It exists as the monovalent fluoride anion F$^-$. This is the only form of interest in nutrition. It is a member of the halogen group and other members of the group include chlorine Cl, bromine Br, and iodine I.

## Biological Functions

- In the body fluorine occurs as calcium fluoride which is found predominantly in bones and teeth where it may act as a strengthening agent. It seems that it helps teeth to resist the action of organisms that cause decay. In teeth, it may also contribute to the white appearance of the tooth. In bone, it increases the density which could be beneficial in offsetting some brittle bone conditions.

- In some laboratory animals, it has been found that traces of fluoride enhance the growth rate. The significance of this effect in humans is unknown.

- There is also indirect evidence that fluoride may be an essential element. The level of fluoride in the blood plasma and soft tissues is regulated within narrow limits.

- The overall level of fluoride in the body tends to increase with age. Values in bone range typically from about 20 to 50 mg per 100 grams of bone, and may rise to much higher levels in some cases.

## Requirement

Fluoride distribution in food and water varies widely depending on the soil content and location. Typical adult intakes of fluoride vary from about 1 to 2 mg per day in non-fluoridated areas and up to about 4 mg per day in areas with a fluoridated tap water supply. The recommended optimum fluoride concentration in drinking water is about 1 mg per litre in temperate climates. The recommended adult daily intake of fluoride in males is 4.0 mg/d and in females it is 3.0 mg/d, respectively.

Considerable controversy still surrounds the whole issue of fluoride in nutrition and health. It has been argued that fluoride toothpaste together with correct eating habits should be sufficient to prevent dental caries and therefore there should be no need to supplement fluoride intake by treating the water supply. Nevertheless, concentrations in drinking water are carefully monitored and adjusted to take account of the natural level of fluoride from place to place. As a general rule, it has been shown that a standard 1 mg fluoride per litre of drinking water is not only safe but also beneficial. Because normal amounts obtained from food alone may vary from as little as 0.3 mg to over ten times that amount per day, depending on geographical location, this recommendation seems reasonable. But the fact that adults cannot incorporate extra fluoride into their teeth once they are formed, together with the observation that some children develop mottled teeth when their drinking water contained 2 to 8 mg fluoride per litre, leaves room for further research.

A fluoride compendium is included for reference (Table 38.1). About 90 percent of fluoride in food is absorbed in the small intestine and is excreted mainly in the urine. Apart from drinking water, tea itself is a major source of fluoride. Three ordinary cups of tea can supply about 1 mg fluoride. Strong tea supplies even more than this. Most of our fluoride comes from beverages, which typically supply up to 77 percent of our requirement. Grain products supply about 10 percent and meat, fish and seafood a further 7 percent, on average.

## Toxicity

Fluoride is a potentially toxic element in relatively small amounts, and its effects may be cumulative. Fluoride causes the enamel of teeth to become dull and chalky at high concentrations. In some animals, the teeth become soft and are rapidly worn away. In other animals, the incisors do not wear down (for the opposite reason) and thus they grow too long. Fluoride toxicity also causes retarded growth, poor lactation and reproductive problems possibly through an appetite suppressant action.

In very high concentrations, fluoride may inhibit certain enzymes, including the energy releasing enzyme ATPase, and the phosphate releasing enzyme alkaline phosphatase, as well as some enzymes involved in carbohydrate and lipid metabolism. Prolonged intakes of fluoride in the range 20 to 80 mg per day eventually produce toxic symptoms such as fluorosis (discolouration and pitting of teeth), osteosclerosis and possibly even cancer.

## Deficiency

Apparently, there are no convincing deficiency symptoms in humans apart from the increased incidence of dental caries, especially in children who do not have fluoride in their drinking water or who do not brush their teeth regularly with a fluoride containing toothpaste.

**Table 38.1.** Fluoride compendium

| FOOD GROUP | FLUORIDE LEVEL |
| --- | --- |
| Milk / Products | Very low / Medium |
| Eggs | Medium |
| Meat / | Medium, variable / |
| Fish | Very high, variable |
| Fats and oils | Medium, variable |
| Grain and products | Very low |
| Nuts and pulses | Low |
| Root vegetables | Very low |
| Leaf vegetables | Very low, variable |
| Fruit | Very low, variable |
| Sweets | Very low, variable |

# 39

# MANGANESE

## Common Name

Manganese (elemental), (Mn).

## Alternative Names

Manganous ion ($Mn^{2+}$).
Manganic ion ($Mn^{3+}$).
Trace Element.

## Nature

Manganese is classified as a transition metal in the d-block, group 7 (VIIA), period 4, of the periodic table of elements. It is a transition element of the first series. It may exist in several oxidation states varying from Mn(II) to Mn(VII). The most common forms include the manganous cation $Mn^{2+}$, and the manganic cation $Mn^{3+}$. Both of these cations occur as active components in certain enzymes and, in some cases, may be interconverted during reactions. These are the only forms presently of interest in nutrition.

## Biological Functions

- Some 12 to 20 mg manganese occurs in the human body. Manganese is found mainly in the bone, liver, muscle and skin. At the cellular level, manganese occurs in high concentrations in the mitochondria.

- Manganese serves as a component of certain metal containing enzymes, many of which are found in the mitochondria. These include decarboxylases which remove carboxyl (-COOH) groups, transferases which assist the transfer of small groups from one molecule to another, hydrolases which split up large molecules into smaller fragments for further metabolism, and kinases which are involved in a number of key cellular reactions involving high-energy phosphate groups. Although many of these enzymes may have a non-specific relationship with manganese. One of the best-known functions of manganese is its role in the activation of enzymes involved in glycoprotein formation and metabolism. This group of substances includes the oligosaccharides, the proteoglycans and the glycoproteins, which are related.

- Recently it has been found that manganese particularly with choline supplements, may act to mobilise fatty deposits in the liver and skin in certain animals. The role of manganese in this effect is not yet known. Nor is it known whether the same effect can be used therapeutically in humans.

- Schizophrenics may benefit from supplements of manganese which may help displace copper from the body. Schizophrenics have been found to have relatively high levels of copper in their bodies.

- Manganese may improve the utilisation of iron and offset certain forms of anaemia.

- Manganese may have a therapeutic effect on the rare nerve disease myasthenia gravis, which is a disturbance of acetylcholine receptor activity.

## Requirement

Manganese values are known to be highly variable. Manganese has not been studied in great detail because a deficiency is extremely rare in humans. For this reason, the food values of manganese are incomplete at present. A manganese compendium is included for reference (Table 39.1). The recommended adult daily intake of manganese in males is 2.3 mg/d and in females is 1.8 mg/d, respectively, whereas the normal levels of intake are around 5 mg per day.

Manganese appears to be best absorbed from the small intestine by a mechanism which may compete with iron. Low levels of iron enhance manganese uptake whereas high levels of iron can inhibit this uptake. Interestingly, alcohol promotes the absorption of manganese. Overall, only some 3 to 5 percent of the manganese in the diet is actually absorbed. Tea is a very rich source of manganese. A single cup of strong tea may provide up to 1 mg manganese. Refined grains are relatively poor in manganese. But tea traditionally makes up for this by providing typically up to 3 mg per day on average. Most of our manganese comes from various beverages which may supply some 56 percent of our requirement. A further 27 percent is obtained from grain products, and about 10 percent comes from various fruit and vegetables.

The main route of excretion of manganese is through the bile and hence the faeces. About 4 mg per day is lost in the faeces, although most of this manganese represents the unabsorbed portion of the diet.

## Toxicity

Manganese has a relatively low toxicity in humans. Dietary intakes up to 15 per day do not produce toxic symptoms. Industrial exposure to manganese ores (particularly those containing the divalent form $Mn^{2+}$), during processing or mining however may result in toxic symptoms. Excessive amounts of manganese are secreted in the bile which is formed in the liver. This is a mechanism which helps to regulate the amount of manganese in the body. The main symptoms of toxicity include a number of complaints relating to the control of muscle movements and posture, lethargy and even coma. Severe toxicity may result in mental disturbances known as manganese madness.

## Deficiency

In experimental animals, a deficiency of manganese may result in poor skeletal development, and disturbances of sexual development including the ability to reproduce. In humans, it has been observed that the manganese levels in the blood of diabetics is only about half the normal value. In a number of other diseases, the blood levels of manganese have also been discovered to be lower than normal; these include heart disease, atherosclerosis and arthritic conditions, schizophrenia and myasthenia gravis. It is not clear yet how to interpret these findings.

Lack of manganese may also affect certain enzymes that require the metal as a catalyst. Excess of iron, calcium or phosphorous in the diet may reduce the absorption of manganese from the diet. Manganese deficiency in certain animals has a specific effect in reducing the activity of a liver enzyme called arginase. This enzyme converts the amino acid arginine to ornithine, with the formation of urea. In certain individuals, deficiency of manganese may lead to anaemia. In fowl, chick perosis is caused by manganese deficiency.

**Table 39.1.** Manganese compendium

| FOOD GROUP | MANGANESE LEVEL |
|---|---|
| Milk and produce | Nil |
| Eggs | Medium |
| Meat and fish | Nil, variable |
| Fats and oils | Nil |
| Grain and products | Very high, variable |
| Nuts and pulses | Very high, variable |
| Root vegetables | Medium, variable |
| Leaf vegetables | High, variable |
| Fruit | High, variable |
| Sweets | Nil |

# 40

# COPPER

## Common Name

Copper (elemental), (Cu).

## Alternative Name

*Cuprum.*
Cuprous ion ($Cu^+$). Cupric ion ($Cu^{2+}$).
Trace Element.

## Nature

Copper is classified as a transition metal in the d-block, group 11 (IB), period 4, of the periodic table of elements. It is a member of the first transition series. It occurs mainly as the divalent cupric cation $Cu^{2+}$ (which is predominantly blue), but also as the monovalent cuprous cation $Cu^+$ (which is predominantly red). These arise from the oxidation states Cu(II) and Cu(I), respectively. The symbol Cu comes from the Latin word for copper namely *cuprum.*

## Biological Functions

- In 1928 copper was shown to be one of the essential trace elements. Copper being a transition metal acts as a component of oxidation-reduction enzymes called oxidoreductases.

- Copper acts together with iron in the formation of haemoglobin in the red blood cell. Specifically, it acts by maturing the cell and by prolonging its life-span. It is not part of the haemoglobin molecule itself.

- Copper acts to maintain the integrity of the nerve cell cover called myelin. Copper is involved in bone and connective tissue, and it also has a role in the formation of skin and hair pigmentation. The pigment melanin is formed from the amino acid tyrosine. Copper is involved in the process called keratinisation.

- Copper occurs as a component of several protein and enzyme systems. It is known to occur in association with cytochrome c oxidase, tyrosinase, uricase, amine oxidase, methionine synthase and dopamine beta-hydroxylase, which are important catalysts in the body. Also, it inhibits the action of amylase, the starch-splitting enzyme.

- In blood plasma, 80 percent of the copper is carried by a special protein called ceruloplasmin. The remaining 20 percent is loosely bound to albumin, the main plasma protein.

- Approximately the same amount of copper occurs inside the red blood cells as occurs in the plasma. In the red cell, most of the copper is bound to a substance called erythrocuprein ($Cu_2Zn_2$ superoxide dismutase). Erythrocuprein protects the cell against dangerous levels of superoxide anions. It catalyses the conversion of superoxide, $O_2^-$, and hydrogen, $H^+$, to oxygen, $O_2$, and hydrogen peroxide, $H_2O_2$.

- Copper is involved in the production of nucleic acids in the body.

- Copper may have a slight anti-inflammatory effect, particularly in association with certain pain killers.

- Copper acts somewhat like an antibiotic in certain animal diets. Minute traces of copper added to feedstuffs promote the growth of pigs and chickens, for example, but this effect is not applicable to humans.

## Requirement

The recommended adult daily intake of copper in both males and in females is 900 µg/d. Some diets provide about 1 mg per day, therefore copper deficiency is possible but unlikely. The liver is a major store of copper. Up to 4 percent of the daily intake of copper is lost in the urine, but the main losses occurs in the faeces.

Copper is very widely distributed in food. A copper compendium is included for reference (Table 40.1). Food processing and storage methods can increase the copper content in the diet. Copper pipes and kettles can increase the copper content of drinking water. Meat and fish supply up to 27 percent of our copper requirement and grain and grain products supply a further 26 percent on average. Vegetables contribute about 18 percent and fruit adds another 14 percent.

## Toxicity

Copper is a potentially toxic element in relatively small amounts. Acute symptoms of copper toxicity may include, low blood pressure, black "tarry faeces, coma, jaundice, gastrointestinal distress and hematemesis (vomiting of blood). Long-term effects include liver and kidney damage. People with glucose-6-phosphate deficiency may be at increased risk of haematological effects of copper toxicity. As it happens, some symptoms of toxicity are similar to those of a copper deficiency.

In humans, a rare genetic disorder called Wilson's disease results in an excessive retention of copper particularly in the liver and brain due to a lack of the plasma copper carrier called ceruloplasmin. This may result in cirrhosis of the liver and mental disturbances. Another very similar condition is termed Indian childhood cirrhosis. Elevated free copper levels have been observed in Alzheimer's disease.

Increasing the intake of zinc and even iron may help protect against copper toxicity. Increased molybdenum also appears to counteract copper toxicity, at lease in sheep. Alternatively, increased levels of copper may cause a depletion of zinc in the body. In some animals, copper poisoning results in kidney damage.

Copper in water supply pipes can contribute relatively high concentrations of copper to the drinking water. Copper can be higher in hot water taps which should not be used for drinking. High blood concentrations of copper have been found in patients with high blood pressure and in smokers. Symptoms of copper intoxication include nausea, vomiting and diarrhoea. Also, there may be muscle and stomach cramps. In extreme cases, there may be mental confusion and even coma.

## Deficiency

Copper is widespread and a dietary deficiency in humans is rare. A deficiency of copper may result in anaemia. The chief characteristic of copper deficiency anaemia is the occurrence of smaller than normal red blood cells leading to a condition which is termed microcytic anaemia. Interestingly, the overall requirement for copper is ten to twelve times less than that for iron itself. Consequently, many forms of anaemia respond to iron supplements alone (or in combination with certain vitamins), as there is usually sufficient copper present in the diet. Also, copper is stored in the liver and to a lesser extent in certain other organs such as the brain, kidneys, heart and bone marrow.

Some elements such as fluoride, zinc, molybdenum (with sulphate) and calcium if present in high concentrations appear to increase the rate of loss of copper from the body and may thus indirectly cause a deficiency. Infants must generally rely on their stores of copper at birth which serve as a reserve before they are weaned, because milk itself is relatively deficient in copper. Infants who are deficient in copper may develop diarrhoea and brittle bones. Menke's syndrome is a rare genetic disorder affecting boys which results in poor transport of copper across the placenta before birth. Such infants develop a steely-haired appearance. Other factors which tend to decrease the copper level in the body include the antibiotic penacillamine and some illnesses. Some patients with heart disease have been found to have lowered copper levels, but the significance of this observation is not yet certain.

One result of copper deficiency is a loss of hair colour which is most noticeable in people with black hair which turns grey. Also, the skin may become very pale the sense of taste may be affected. Disturbances of copper have also been seen in patients with rheumatoid arthritis. Interestingly, copper can be absorbed through the skin from copper bracelets for example, and this may well form the basis for the belief that such items if worn regularly can cure some arthritic conditions.

In some animals, a deficiency of copper tends to elevate the blood cholesterol levels. Swayback syndrome results in lambs, if the net copper accumulation in the body is inadequate. Falling disease in cattle is similar condition. Certain pastures rich in molybdenum but low in copper may result in a condition termed peat scours, and sudden death may occur due to heart failure. In sheep, the normal crimping of the wool does not occur and its rate of growth is decreased. In addition, normally black wool may turn white, and in some cases, there may be wool loss. In other animals, a wide variety of specific symptoms have been documented. Cardiovascular changes are frequent in many animals, elastic membranes such as the aorta may be weakened due to lack of synthesis of the protein called elastin which is essential for these structures.

**Table 40.1.** Copper compendium

| FOOD GROUP | COPPER LEVEL |
| --- | --- |
| Milk / Products | Nil / High, variable |
| Eggs | Very low |
| Meat and fish | Very variable |
| Fats and oils | Nil, variable |
| Grain and products | Medium |
| Nuts and pulses | High, variable |
| Root vegetables | Low |
| Leaf vegetables | Low |
| Fruit | Low |
| Sweets | Nil |

# 41

## IODINE

### Common Name

Iodine (elemental, not gaseous), (I, not $I_2$).

### Alternative Names

Iodide ion ($I^-$).
Organic and Inorganic Iodine.
Trace Element.

### Nature

Iodine is classified as a nonmetal in the p-block, group 17 (VIIB), period 5, of the periodic table of elements. It is member of the halogen group. Other members of this group include fluorine F, chlorine Cl, and bromine Br. It exists as either iodine (often organically bound) or as the monovalent iodide anion $I^-$. As both the atomic and the ionic forms are common, the term iodide has been used generically to include both forms which are interconvertible in the body. Most of the iodine in the diet is absorbed as iodide.

### Biological Functions

- Before 1900, a lack of iodine was known to be the cause of goitre. Iodine was the second element after iron to be recognised as essential. Seaweed was discovered to contain iodine as long ago as 1811. In 1820, Coindet first used seaweed to treat goitre in humans. In 1895 Baumann detected iodine in the thyroid gland.

- Iodine is the only mineral which becomes incorporated into the essential structure of a hormone. About 25 percent of the iodine in the human body is found in the thyroid gland. Its sole recognised function in the human body is its role in the formation of the thyroid hormones. These hormones regulate a wide variety of systems involved in cell development and metabolic rate. They act by regulating a very large number of enzymes, involved in growth, reproduction, metabolism and energy supply.

- In the thyroid gland, iodine uptake is promoted by the thyroid stimulating hormone (TSH) of the pituitary gland in the brain. Iodide is oxidised to iodine and incorporated into thyroglobulin by iodination of tyrosine residues. Tyrosine may combine with one or two iodine atoms to form either mono-, or di-, iodotyrosine. These occur in approximately equal amounts except during iodine deficiency when the mono- form predominates. Two molecules of diiodotyrosine may combine to form the hormone called thyroxine (which is chemically termed tetraiodothyronine), or $T_4$ for short. If one molecule of the mono-form and one molecule of the di- form combine, the result is a related hormone called triiodothyronine, or $T_3$. The $T_3$ form is about four times more biologically active than the $T_4$ form. In the body, $T_4$ can also be converted to $T_3$, after it is formed. There are two distinct chemical forms of $T_3$. In general, all the biologically active forms are loosely referred to as Thyroid Hormone. Most of the thyroid hormones circulating in the body are bound to proteins. Only a small fraction is free and hence biologically active. Also, in the thyroid, hormones are metabolised to acidic forms which are only about one-fourth as active as their precursors.

- Iodine is found in muscle tissue, salivary glands, parts of the eye and in the ovaries. But its role, if any, in these tissues is unknown.

- Iodine is found in milk and is transferred to the young by this route.

- Iodine has several biological properties; it has antioxidant, anti-inflammatory, pro-differentiating, and pro-apoptotic effects. These roles can play a part in preventing cancer, particularly stomach and breast cancers. Other cancers are under investigation at present, including prostate cancer, endometrial, ovarian, colorectal, and thyroid cancers. It is not clear whether these are due to a hypothyroid state, autoimmune processes or iodine deficiency per se.

## Requirement

The iodine content of various foods is highly variable depending on the soil conditions. The only consistently high source of iodine is in various seafoods, as can be seen in the accompanying compendium (Tables 41.1). The minimum adult requirement of iodine is about 1 µg per kg of body weight per day. This amount represents some 50 to 75 µg per day, and is sufficient to prevent goitre. The recommended adult daily intake of iodine in both males and in females is 150 µg/d. Additional amounts are required during pregnancy and lactation.

The safe intake level of iodine is considered to be in the range up to 1 mg per day. Iodine occurs in several forms in food. The inorganic form called iodide, I⁻, is readily absorbed because it is assisted by an active transport process. In fact, iodide is virtually completely absorbed from the diet but over half is rapidly excreted in the urine. Most of the remainder is concentrated in the thyroid gland. The average adult intake of iodine in the Western diet varies from about 250 to 85 µg per day, but the intake for individuals also varies widely from day to day.

As a general recommendation, it has been suggested that wherever salt is used in the diet it should preferably contain some iodine. Iodide salt contains around 76 µg iodine per gram of salt. Bearing in mind the comments made in the Chapter on sodium regarding salt intake, just 2 grams of iodide salt would provide the full daily requirement for iodine.

Some average values of iodine are given in micrograms per 100 grams as follows: seafood, various 65; vegetables, 25; meat and eggs, 20; cheese, various, 15; bread, 10; fruit, 5; and milk, 2, respectively. In contrast iodide salt contains 76 µg per gram and drinking water contains only minute traces depending on the area. About 36 percent of our iodine requirement comes from milk and its products. Meat and especially fish supply a further 20 percent on average. Grain and products supply about 12 percent, fruit another 10 percent, and vegetables about 9 percent.

## Toxicity

Iodine is not toxic in amounts available from food. Supplements containing iodine may however lead to toxicity, if overused. Oral solutions, such as Lugol's iodine, can cause temporary burning of the mouth and throat. Excessive iodine intake may depress thyroid activity. Symptoms of iodine toxicity include, fever, nausea, vomiting, diarrhoea, a weak pulse, cyanosis, and ultimately coma.

## Deficiency

A deficiency of iodine the diet leads to an enlargement of the thyroid gland (in the neck) called goitre. This enlargement can be very extensive depending on the degree of deficiency. A large number of people suffer from a mild form of goitre depending on their geographical location. About 1 µg per kg body weight is sufficient to prevent goitre.

High levels of certain metals such manganese and cobalt can interfere with iodine uptake by the thyroid gland. Certain natural substances in foods, particularly the vegetables of the Brassica family such as cabbage and turnips, cause this effect. These substances are called goitrogens. Large intakes of Brassicas over an extended period of time are not therefore advisable. Milk from animals fed on Brassicas may also contain the goitrogens and therefore if taken in large amounts can also be harmful. During pregnancy and lactation, iodine requirements are increased. Infants who fail to get enough iodine develop cretinism which is characterised by stunted growth and poor mental development. Other symptoms in children include deaf mutism. Adolescent girls often develop symptoms of iodine deficiency due to generalised hormonal changes during that time and just before menstruation. There is some evidence that a lack of iodine in some women may predispose them towards the development of cancer of the womb.

**Table 41.1.** Iodine compendium

| FOOD GROUP | IODINE LEVEL |
| --- | --- |
| Milk / Products | Very low / Medium, variable |
| Eggs | Medium, variable |
| Meat / Fish | Medium, variable / Very high |
| Fats and oils | Very variable |
| Grain and products | Low |
| Nuts and pulses | Low |
| Root vegetables | Medium, variable |
| Leaf vegetables | Medium, variable |
| Fruit | Very low |
| Sweets | Nil |

# 42

## SELENIUM

### Common Name

Selenium (elemental), (Se).

### Alternative Name

Trace element.

### Nature

Selenium Se, is classified as a nonmetal in the p-block, group 16 (VIA), period 4, of the periodic table of elements. It is found in the same group as oxygen O, and sulphur S. Selenium occurs in several forms and it may exhibit several oxidation states. It may occur as elemental selenium Se, selenide $Se^{2-}$, selenite $SeO^{3-}$, or it may be organically bound as selenosulphide derivatives.

### Biological Functions

- Selenium is one of the most recently recognised essential trace elements. Although it was not until the seventies that the major interest in selenium commenced, the first indicators of its importance were discovered by Klaus Schwartz in 1957.

- In human males, about 50 percent of the selenium in the body is found in the testes and seminal glands.

- Selenium can offset some symptoms of vitamin E deficiency. Selenium, like vitamin E, is an antioxidant. Vitamin C and zinc also have antioxidant properties.

- Selenium is involved in the enzymatic synthesis of certain prostaglandins

- It has been found that the incidence of heart disease is lower where the average selenium intake in the diet is higher. Also, selenium may ameliorate some cases of high blood pressure. Selenium counteracts the effects of certain heavy metals such as cadmium which may cause a form of high blood pressure by accumulating in the kidney.

- Selenium may be involved in regulating the levels of Coenzyme Q (CoQ or ubiquinone), which is found in greater concentrations in heart tissue than in any other type of muscle.

- Together with vitamin E, selenium may help to relieve the pain of angina.

- People living in areas with selenium rich soils have a lower incidence of cancer. It has been shown that the higher the average concentration of selenium is, in the blood plasma, the lower the average death rate is, from many types of cancer.

- Selenium may be beneficial in the treatment of certain forms of arthritis.

- Selenium acts cooperatively with vitamin E to counteract the biologically harmful effects of free radicles. This may be the molecular basis for many of the observations attributed to selenium, including an apparent slowing of the ageing process in certain cases.

- Many of the above observations are under intensive research at present.

## Requirement

The selenium content of food varies widely according to the soil conditions. Some agricultural areas are in fact deficient in selenium. The average intake of dietary selenium is about 150 µg per day in most areas of the United States. In contrast, certain areas in Italy yield a total daily intake of only one-tenth of this value, whereas Venezuela yields about twice this value. The selenium content of drinking water likewise varies from about 1 to 50 µg per litre, depending on location. It is clear therefore that a deficiency of selenium is a possibility in certain areas.

A dietary intake of 20 to 30 micrograms per day is probably sufficient to maintain selenium balance. The recommended adult daily intake of selenium in both males and in females is 55 µg/d. In general, it should be noted that fruit and vegetables are very poor sources of selenium and are insufficient in themselves to maintain the recommended intakes. Yeast, garlic, mushrooms and radishes are rich sources of selenium. About half of our selenium requirement comes from grain products. A further 37 percent normally comes from meat and fish. A selenium compendium is included for reference (Table 42.1).

## Toxicity

It is not generally advisable to supplement the daily intake of selenium with more than about 200 µg on a regular basis, although intakes over 1,000 µg per day appear to be safe. Interestingly, in Japan where fishermen eat fish every day, the estimated daily intake has been calculated to be about 5,000 µg, with no toxic side effects. Nevertheless, selenium is a potentially toxic element in relatively small amounts. Symptoms of intoxication include gastrointestinal disorders and lung irritation. Other symptoms include a smell of garlic on the breath, loss of hair and nails and various nervous disturbances.

Sodium selenite is a very toxic form of selenium and has been replaced by selenium rich yeast as the main oral supplementary form. A single dose of 1,000 µg of the selenite form may produce toxic symptoms in certain individuals, whereas the same dose of the yeast form which is organically bound selenium should not produce toxic symptoms as it is only one-third as toxic as the inorganic form. Selenium sulphide is also very toxic and is not intended for internal use, but it acts as a treatment for dandruff or dermatitis of the scalp when used in shampoos.

## Deficiency

Lack of selenium can cause damage to the heart, kidneys and liver. Also, in certain laboratory animals, a deficiency had been shown to interfere with reproduction. There may also be an increased risk of developing atherosclerosis, heart disease, cancer and related diseases. Low levels of selenium have been found in patients with cystic fibrosis, but it is too early to interpret the significance of these findings. In lambs, a lack of selenium and vitamin E may lead to a form of muscular dystrophy. However, the same may not hold true for humans, although there is some evidence that a link may be present. Low levels of selenium increase the risk of damage caused by pollution and radiation to the body, reduce the general resistance to disease and may result in impaired healing of wounds.

**Table 42.1.** Selenium compendium

| FOOD GROUP | SELENIUM LEVEL |
| --- | --- |
| Milk / Products | Low / High |
| Eggs | High |
| Meat and fish | Very high, variable |
| Fats and oils | Very low |
| Grain and products | Very high, variable |
| Nuts and pulses | Very low |
| Root vegetables | Very low, variable |
| Leaf vegetables | Low, variable |
| Fruit | Very low |
| Sweets | Very low, variable |

# 43

# MOLYBDENUM

## Common Name

Molybdenum (elemental), (Mo).

## Alternative Name

Trace element.

## Nature

Molybdenum is classified as a transition metal in the d-block, group 6 (VIA), period 5, of the periodic table of elements. Being a transition element of the second series, it is one of the few heavy metals known to be essential for life. Molybdenum occurs in the same group as chromium. It may exist in several oxidation states, but the most stable of these Mo(VI), is exhibited by the molybdate anion, $MoO_4^{2-}$. Some other oxidation states, varying from Mo(II) to Mo(V), may exist during certain enzyme reactions in which molybdenum is actively involved. The essential function of molybdenum as a cofactor for the enzyme xanthine oxidase was discovered in 1953 by De Renzo, *et al.*

## Biological Functions

* Molybdenum is a cofactor for three separate enzymes, namely xanthine oxidase, aldehyde oxidase and sulphite oxidase.

* The enzymes, xanthine oxidase is perhaps the best-known example. This enzyme is involved in the breakdown of nucleic acid purine bases to yield uric acid. Uric acid is very insoluble and tends to form stones if present in excessive amounts. It may also lead to gout in susceptible individuals. Xanthine oxidase also

acts on some aldehydes and pterins.

- Molybdenum may be involved, again through the enzyme xanthine oxidase, in making iron available in the body from certain food components.

- Molybdenum assists the breakdown of toxic sulphites and helps fight cancer-causing nitrosamines.

- It has been suggested but not yet proved that molybdenum may help to prevent dental caries.

- Molybdenum helps to maintain the normal sexual function in the male.

- A high amount of molybdenum in the body could interfere with the absorption of copper and can cause a fatal deficiency. Alternatively, high concentrations, molybdenum may help to remove excess copper from the body.

## Requirement

The molybdenum values for many foods are not fully known. The content is highly variable and depends on the soil. The compendium indicates some typical levels of molybdenum but these should be considered as approximate (Table 43.1). Molybdenum levels vary from 120 to 20 µg per litre in cow's milk. Milk, fruit and root vegetables, most muscle meats and eggs are poor sources of molybdenum. Pulses are a very rich source. Dry products, certain leafy vegetables, and liver and kidney are also rich sources.

It is highly improbable that molybdenum deficiency occurs in humans as only minute traces are required and these are widely distributed. The average intake of molybdenum in the Western diet has been estimated to range from 120 to 240 µg per day, and this is sufficient to maintain a positive molybdenum balance. The recommended adult daily intake of molybdenum in both males and in females is 45 µg/d. Molybdenum is absorbed from the intestines and stored in the liver, bones and kidneys. About half of the molybdenum in the diet is absorbed and the main route of excretion is in the urine.

## Toxicity

In humans, excessive intake of molybdenum, somewhere in the range around 15 mg per day, can inhibit certain enzymes and may result in gout. However, the normal intake is generally less than 2 mg per day in most areas. A high amount of molybdenum in the body could interfere with the absorption of copper and can even cause a fatal deficiency. Alternatively, high concentrations, molybdenum may help to remove excess copper from the body.

Molybdenum is a potentially toxic element in relatively small amounts. Some soils contain levels of molybdenum sufficient to cause toxicity in cattle and sheep which appear to be the most susceptible domestic animals. The chief symptoms of molybdenum intoxication in animals include severe diarrhoea, loss of appetite and anaemia. There is also poor growth in young animals. The severity of the symptoms however, depend on the levels of copper and sulphur also in the diet. In some animals, there may be dermatitis, loss of hair, decreased lactation and even male sterility.

## Deficiency

As stated above a deficiency of molybdenum in humans is highly improbable. Certain soils are very low in molybdenum, especially soils which are relatively rich in copper. Deficiency results in defects in uric acid production, sulphur amino acid metabolism and sulphite sensitivity. Sulphite oxidase deficiency may lead to neurological damage. Gross molybdenum deficiency may lead to irritability, headaches, night blindness, rapid heartbeat, rapid respiration and even coma.

**Table 43.1.** Molybdenum compendium

| FOOD GROUP | MOLYBDENUM LEVEL |
| --- | --- |
| Milk and products | Very low |
| Eggs | Low |
| Meat and fish | Very variable |
| Fats and oils | Nil |
| Grain and products | Very high |
| Nuts and pulses | Very high |
| Root vegetables | Very low |
| Leaf vegetables | Medium, variable |
| Fruit | Very low |
| Sweets | Very low, variable |

# 44

# CHROMIUM

## Common Name

Chromium (elemental), (Cr).

## Alternative Name

Trace element.

## Nature

Chromium is generally classified as a transition metal in the d-block, group 6 (VIA), period 4, of the periodic table of elements. It is a member of the first transition series. Chromium therefore exists in several oxidation states, the most common being Cr(III), giving rise to the stable trivalent cation $Cr^{3+}$. Other oxidation states varying from Cr(II) to Cr(VI) exist but are probably not important nutritionally. Hexavalent Cr(VI) is toxic and carcinogenic. Chromium was shown to be an essential trace element by Schroeder, *et al.*, around 1968. It is therefore one of the most recently recognised essential nutrients.

## Biological Functions

- Chromium aids insulin action and glucose metabolism. The trivalent form of chromium plays an important role in carbohydrate metabolism. A complex called the glucose tolerance factor (GTF) contains chromium and acts to control the blood glucose level. The glucose tolerance factor forms a complex in cellular membranes involving the hormone insulin which is the main hormone promoting the uptake of glucose by the cells.

- Chromium plays a role in the metabolism of lipids. Chromium stimulates fatty acid and cholesterol synthesis, which is important for brain function and other body processes. In experimental animals, chromium is known to reduce the level of cholesterol in the blood.

- Chromium also has a role to play in protein metabolism. It may help to incorporate the dietary amino acids into protein in muscles including the heart. This aspect of chromium metabolism in under intensive investigation at present.

- Chromium stimulates the production of certain nerve transmitters in the body.

- Serotonin (also called 5-hydroxytryptamine, 5-HT) is a neurotransmitter derived from tryptophan. Serotonin receptors are widely distributed in the central nervous system and modulate the release of many sympathetic and parasympathetic neurotransmitters, including gamma-aminobutyric acid (GABA), dopamine, noradrenaline, and acetylcholine. Chromium can modify brain (5-HT) function in humans and animals, perhaps by altering the sensitivity of central $5\text{-HT}_{2A}$ receptors.

- Chromium picolinate (400 µg/d) may have antidepressant properties, perhaps through increasing the peripheral availability of tryptophan for synthesis of serotonin (5-HT) in the brain.

- Chromium decreases the sensitivity of type 2A 5-HT receptors.

- Chromium lowers the cortisol response to challenge with 5-hydroxytryptophan (5-HTP) in humans and rats.

- Chromium may increase the resistance to various infections.

## Requirement

It has been found the chromium intake in the range 20 to 45 µg per day is sufficient to maintain chromium balance. The recommended adult daily intake of chromium in males is 35 µg/d and in females is 25 µg/d, respectively. Average intakes in Western diets are several times higher than this, being typically 90 to 150 µg per day, and in some cases, up to 4 mg per day. Nevertheless, the possibility of chromium deficiency does occasionally occur, because only around

10 percent of dietary chromium is absorbed. The body content of chromium is highest at birth and falls with age. There may be an additional requirement for chromium during pregnancy and lactation. In certain experimental animals, supplements of chromium are known to improve growth and increase the life-span.

The chromium distribution in various foods is highly variable depending on the soil. Brewer's yeast, nuts, shell fish, free range eggs, grass-fed beef, liver, and some fruit and vegetables are good sources of chromium. The compendium indicates some typical levels of chromium (Table 44.1). Natural foods such as molasses, honey, whole grain bread and brown rice, contain much more chromium than refined foods such as white bread, white rice and sugar. Drinking water usually contains very little chromium but in places it may contain around 1 μg per litre. Significant amounts of chromium can arise from cooking in stainless steel utensils.

Over a day, the average adult will lose some 7 to 12 μg of chromium, mostly in the urine with some also in the faeces. Chromium is best absorbed in organic combination in the form called glucose tolerance factor. Trivalent chromium can improve the glucose tolerance of patients suffering from protein-energy malnutrition. After a sugar meal both the insulin and the chromium levels in the blood are observed to rise. Inorganic chromium is very poorly absorbed. Typically, only 1 percent of the inorganic form is absorbed. Therefore, diets cannot be satisfactorily evaluated at present because the ratio of the organic to the inorganic forms of chromium which determine the overall rate of uptake are not all known. It is believed that chromium shares an uptake mechanism with zinc in the small intestine. Chromium is stored in the tissues. It is transported to the tissues by transferrin which also carries iron. Much of the chromium occurs in the mitochondria especially in the liver.

## Toxicity

Dietary toxicity of chromium is extremely rare. Most cases of chromium toxicity arise because of industrial contamination in the form of chromium dust. The hexavalent form of chromium, Cr(VI), is much more toxic than the trivalent form, Cr(III). Chronic inhalation of Cr(VI) can cause pulmonary sensitization and increase the risk of lung cancer. Severe dermatitis and skin ulcers can also result from contact with Cr(VI) compounds. Doses of Cr(VI) above 1 gram in humans can be fatal.

Cr(VI) is rapidly reduced to Cr(III) in the gastric juice and also after entering cells. Cr(VI) can be readily transported into cells, whereas Cr(III) has much less ability to cross membranes. The reduction of Cr(VI) to Cr(III) inside of cells may contribute to the toxicity of chromium, whereas the reduction of Cr(VI) to Cr(III) outside cells may act as a fortuitous protective mechanism. Even when present in very large quantities, trivalent chromium has little toxic effect. The toxic effects of hexavalent chromium include dermatitis, allergic skin reactions, ulcerations, allergic asthma, bronchial carcinoma, gastroenteritis, and liver and kidney damage.

## Deficiency

A deficiency of chromium may increase the vulnerability to diabetes in adults. Some soils are very poor in chromium. Highly refined and processed foodstuffs may also be deficient in chromium. Chromium is very poorly absorbed from the gut where as much as 97 percent may remain unabsorbed after a meal. Symptoms of deficiency include various nervous complaints, feelings of frustration, poor memory, mental confusion and even depression. There may be a generalised weakness, itching, hunger, thirst, increased blood lipid levels including cholesterol, and weight loss.

High sugar intake may deplete chromium due to the impact of elevated insulin on chromium loss via the urine. The gradual loss of chromium from the body with age has been associated with a form of diabetes which develops in the middle years called maturity onset diabetes. Supplementary chromium may improve this condition in some cases, and levels up to 250 µg per day have been used for this purpose. In certain experimental animals, a chromium deficiency can arise because of repeated pregnancies, if the animals are on a low intake diet. Lack of chromium may result in high cholesterol levels, atherosclerosis, and even heart disease. A deficiency may increase the vulnerability to heart attacks. A lack of chromium may also reduce the ability to tolerate alcohol. This effect is believed to be due to the effect of alcohol in increasing blood sugar. In other words, the effect is strictly not an alcohol intolerance but a glucose intolerance. The effect may be more severe in alcoholics who are on a poor nutritional diet.

**Table 44.1.** Chromium compendium

| FOOD GROUP | CHROMIUM LEVEL |
| --- | --- |
| Milk / Products | Nil / Medium, variable. |
| Eggs | Low, variable |
| Meat and fish | Medium, variable |
| Fats and oils | Nil, variable |
| Grain and product | Medium, variable |
| Nuts and pulses | Medium, variable |
| Root vegetables | Low, variable |
| Leaf vegetables | Medium, variable |
| Fruit | Very low, variable |
| Sweets | Low, variable |

# 45

## Some Lesser-Known Trace and Ultratrace Elements

**Tin, Silicon, Boron, Aluminium, Bromide, Rubidium, Strontium, Barium, Germanium, Lithium, Nickel, Lead, Cadmium, Silver, Arsenic, Vanadium, Gold.**

The nutritional importance of many trace elements is very difficult to prove. The requirements may be so minimal that they are easily met by the natural levels occurring in food and even in drinking water. The strictest laboratory conditions are therefore required to produce deficiency states for some trace elements. Several studies have shown that some lesser known elements appear to be essential in microorganisms, plants or even animals. Much work remains to be done to fully clarify the possible roles of many of these ultratrace elements as potentially essential nutrients in humans. Several these will be briefly considered in this final chapter.

### Tin

Tin Sn, is a post-transition heavy metal in the p-block, Group 14 (IVB), Period 5, of the periodic table of elements. Group 14 also contains carbon, silicon, germanium and lead.

In the sixties, tin was shown to be essential for growth of certain animals. Tin is possibly essential in humans. The functions of tin may include catalysing the synthesis of nucleic acids and proteins. The daily requirements for tin are unknown but an estimated intake of 1 to 3 mg per day is considered to be adequate. High consumption of canned products may contribute significantly to total tin intake and occasionally intakes up to 45 mg per day have been known to occur. The average daily intakes are probable in the range 4 to 16 mg per day. Only a small amount of this is absorbed from the gut.

Tin is toxic at levels greater than about 5 mg per kilogram of body weight. Tin interferes with the metabolism of copper and iron. Tin oxide is occasionally used to treat boils, tapeworms, and similar. In humans, high concentrations of tin cause severe stomach and muscle pain, nausea, constipation, weakness, fever, headaches and ear noises. Tin is also toxic if inhaled as a dust because it may give rise to pneumoconiosis. Toxic effects in animals include anaemia and impaired growth. In some experimental animals, a deficiency of tin retards growth. A deficiency of tin is unknown in humans.

## Silicon

Silicon Si, is a metalloid in the p-block, Group 14 (IVA), Period 5, of the periodic table of elements. Group 14 also contains carbon, germanium, tin and lead.

Silicon is essential for the skeleton structure of certain shellfish and occurs in plants. But it is not clear if humans have an active metabolism of silicon. Silicon in organic linkage is the functional form of the element. Silicon is found in connective tissues, skin, cartilage, tendon, bone and the walls of blood vessels. It was shown in the early seventies by Schwartz and others that silicon occurs in complex carbohydrates called mucopolysaccharides, particularly chondroitin-4-sulphate, dermatin sulphate and heparin sulphate (an anticoagulant) in mammals. These giant molecules contain about one silicon atom per 200 monosaccharide repeating units. The silicon atoms may form links or bridges between different polysaccharide chains.

Silicon markedly increases the collagen in growing bones. In rats and chicks, deficiency of silicon produces deformities of bones and joints and a reduced content of hexosamine and collagen in cartilage. Large doses of silicon may reduce atherosclerosis in cholesterol-fed rabbits. Silicon is involved in the early stages of normal skeletal development of rats and birds. However, it's role in humans is not yet established.

The average intake of silicon is about 0.7 milligrams per 100 grams of mixed food or 2 to 5 mg per day. Only about 5 percent of this is absorbed, but the daily requirement is unknown. Kelp is a rich source of silicon as well as many other trace elements.

Silica (silicon dioxide) is toxic if inhaled as a dust because it may give rise to silicosis. In experimental studies with some animals, a deficiency of silicon can affect growth and the formation of bones. A deficiency of silicon is unknown in humans.

**Boron**

Boron B, is a metalloid in the p-block, Group 13 (IIIB), Period 2, of the periodic table of elements. Group 13 also contains the metal aluminium. Other metalloids include silicon, Germanium and arsenic.

It has been known for a long time that boron is essential for higher plants but apparently not for algae or microorganisms. There is increasing evidence that boron may also be essential for animals. Boron appears to influence calcium and magnesium metabolism. Boron regulates the utilisation of calcium by the bones in humans and strengthens bones by increasing osteoblastic activity, thus minimising the risks of osteoporosis and arthritis. Boron deficiency may be linked to the level of vitamin D in the diet. It may also be needed to maintain the integrity of certain cell membranes, and the normal function of the central nervous system. Other possible symptoms of deficiency include imbalances in the steroid hormones testosterone and estrogen. Hyperthyroidism is another possible symptom. Deficiency of boron may also result in an impaired immune response in higher animals. Deficiency signs have been observed in chickens and rats and also in humans.

**Aluminium**

Aluminium Al, is a post-transition metal in the s-block, group 13 (IIIB), period 3, of the periodic table of elements. Group 13 also contains boron B. Aluminium occurs as a trivalent cation $Al^{3+}$. Group 13 also contains boron.

The biological importance of aluminium is unknown and there are no reports of aluminium deficiency. Most of the aluminium taken up by the human body is excreted.

Aluminium inhibits hexokinase and other enzymes in the brain. Aluminium affects the electrical activity of nerve cells and reduces nervous system activity, and it inhibits the uptake of important neurotransmitters by nerve cells, such as dopamine, noradrenaline and 5-hydroxytryptamine. Aluminium reduces the intestinal activity of smooth muscle cells. Evidence linking aluminium with Alzheimer's disease is circumstantial.

## Bromide

Bromine is classified as a nonmetal in the p-block, group 17 (VIIB), period 4, of the periodic table of elements. It is a member of the halogen group and it exists as the monovalent bromide anion $Br^-$, which is the only form of interest in nutrition. Other elements in group 17 include fluorine, chlorine and iodine. The typical daily intake of bromide is around 2 to 8 mg per day. Bromide is relatively nontoxic.

Recently, an essential role for bromide has been found as a cofactor, enabling peroxidasin to form sulphilimine bonds. Peroxidasin, a haem peroxidase enzyme found in basement membranes, first generates hypobromous acid, BrOH. The enzyme uses hydrogen peroxide, $H_2O_2$, and a bromide ion, $Br^-$, to release a hydroxyl ion, $OH^-$ and generate hypobromous acid, BrOH. The acid can react with the sulphur atom of a methionine to give the following intermediate, $>S^+-Br$. This can go on to form a sulphilimine bond ($>S=N-$) with an amine nitrogen of a hydroxylysine component in another part of the collagen. These sulphilimine cross-links help to stabilise the type IV collagen latticework. Bromide is essential for all animals including humans.

## Rubidium

Rubidium Rb, is an alkali metal in the s-block, group 1 (IA), period 5, of the periodic table of elements. Group 1 also contains lithium, sodium, and potassium.

No specific biological function is known for rubidium. In many respects, rubidium is like potassium, and in some animals, it can replace potassium. Rubidium salts are generally inert. In the body, rubidium can substitute for potassium and large amounts may cause hyperirritability and spasms. Rubidium can replace potassium in the $Na^+/K^+$-ATPase system (sodium-potassium pump). Rubidium chloride has antidepressant activity. Rubidium enhances the release of noradrenaline and may disturb circadian rhythms. No recommended daily allowance has been set for rubidium. The average dietary intake of rubidium is around 1.5 mg/d. It is easily absorbed and eliminated in the urine. There are no known deficiency symptoms for rubidium.

**Strontium and Barium**

Strontium Sr, is an alkaline earth metal in the s-block, group 2 (IIA), period 5, of the periodic table of elements.

Barium Ba, is an alkaline earth metal in the s-block, group 2 (IIA), period 6, of the periodic table of elements.

Group 2 also contains the essential mineral, magnesium.

Strontium and barium may be essential trace elements in some animals. In rats, the omission of either strontium or barium from diets, which were highly purified, caused a depression in growth.

Furthermore, the absence of strontium resulted in impairment of the calcification of the bones and teeth and a higher incidence of dental caries than occurred in control animals.

Interestingly, similar results on the calcification of the bones and teeth were obtained with vanadium.

In contrast to strontium, barium caused decalcification and not mineralization of the osseous tissues.

## Germanium

Germanium Ge, is a metalloid in the s-block, group 14 (IVB), period 4, of the periodic table of elements. Other metalloids include boron B, silicon Si, and arsenic As. Other elements in group 14 include carbon, silicon, tin and lead.

An organic form of germanium, bis-carboxyethyl germanium(IV) sesquioxide, has been tested as a treatment for cancer in a number of trials. Some benefits of germanium have been reported including improvement of the immune system. Germanium helps to neutralise damaging free radicals. Germanium also enhances plant growth.

Germanium may have antioxidant properties and helps reduce inflammation. Germanium has been used for arthritis. It has also been used to treat heavy metal poisoning.

Oral administration of organic germanium induces interferon production. Interferons trigger protective defenses of the immune system and interfere with the replication of viral pathogens. Germanium has a very low toxicity.

## Lithium

Lithium is an alkali metal in the s-block, Group 1 (IA), Period 2, of the periodic table of elements. Group 1 also contains sodium, potassium and rubidium.

Lithium is an alkali metal like potassium and sodium, and it may substitute for sodium and depress nerve conduction. It may exert its action also by decreasing the level of the catecholamines in the brain. Lithium has a pharmacological effect which has been used to relieve both manic and depressive disorders in humans. It is readily absorbed from the gut and is excreted in the urine.

There is a high lithium content in the embryo during early foetal development which may indicate an important role. Lithium can displace magnesium as a cofactor and can inhibit several enzymes, including inositol monophosphatase and glycogen synthase kinase 3. This may be a key to lithium's mechanism of action. In high doses, lithium is toxic and causes kidney damage. It is uncertain whether lithium is nutritionally essential in humans.

## Nickel

Nickel Ni, is a transition metal in the d-block, Group 10 (VIII), Period 4, of the periodic table of elements. Group VIII also contains iron and cobalt. Nickel as Ni(II), is the most common form of the element.

Nickel is known to aid the action of insulin and inhibit the action. of adrenaline. It is believed to be essential for many animals, but its role (if any) in humans in unknown. A function of nickel at the cellular level may be to maintain the integrity of certain membranes. Nickel may play a role in lipid metabolism. Nickel is associated with the enzyme urease which breaks down urea in certain cells. There is a blood protein called nickeloplasmin which contains nickel. Nickel may also stabilise nucleic acids. Nickel promotes the production of red blood cells in some animals.

Nickel is widely distributed in both plants and animals. The daily requirements for nickel are unknown, but a daily intake around 35 µg per day appears adequate. Nickel occurs as a contaminant in hydrogenated vegetable oils including most margarines and peanut butter. It also arises as a contaminant during the preparing and cooking of food in metal utensils.

An upper limit of nickel intake has been established as 1 mg per day. Excessive nickel in the blood is toxic, and been associated with heart attacks, strokes, toxemia and cancer. Nickel carbonyl, which is inhaled in tobacco smoke may be one cause of lung cancer. On the other hand, excessive intakes in food do not generally give rise to toxic effects in humans.

A deficiency of nickel in chickens causes poor growth, thick legs, and dermatitis. In several animals, a deficiency causes swelling of the mitochondria, the key cellular structures required for metabolism and the provision of cellular energy. Deficiency also causes anaemia by impairing iron absorption in certain animals. A deficiency of nickel in humans is unknown, although cirrhosis of the liver is known to be associated with low nickel levels in the blood.

## Lead and Cadmium

Lead Pb, is a post-transition metal in the p-block, Group 14 (IVB), Group 6, of the periodic table of elements. Group 14 also contains carbon, silicon, germanium and tin.

Cadmium Cd, is a metal in the d-block, Group 12 (IIB), Period 5, of the periodic table of elements. Group 12 also contains zinc.

Cadmium and lead are generally classified as heavy metal poisons. They are very toxic and the effects are accumulative. However, that does not rule them out as essential in extremely small amounts.

Depressed growth and poor reproduction have been observed in laboratory animals where cadmium and lead were lacking in the diet. Similar deficiency signs have also been noted when the diets were lacking in tin, lithium and vanadium.

## Silver

Silver Ag, is a metal in the d-block, Group 11 (1B), period 5, of the periodic table of elements. Group 11 also contains copper and gold. Most foods contain traces of silver.

Silver has no biological function and despite its low toxicity, large doses can cause argyria. This condition causes the skin to turn a permanent blue-purple-grey color. However, silver is a good antiseptic and can kill germs on contact. Silver ions $Ag^+$, are deadly to most bacteria, fungi and viruses. A mixture of silver nitrate and potassium nitrate can be used topically to treat warts and verrucae.

Colloidal Silver is a solution of extremely fine nanoparticles (5 - 15 nanometres in diameter) of positively charged pure silver suspended in water. Colloidal silver can be taken orally and is typically recommended at a dosage around 5 µg/kg body weight per day. Initially, there may be a reaction to the silver. The so-called Jarisch-Herxheimer Reaction is a short-term detoxification syndrome, which includes flu-like symptoms, headaches, pains, rashes, sore throat, chills and nausea. During this time, pathogens are being killed off.

## Arsenic

Arsenic As, is a metalloid in the p-block, Group 15 (VB), Period 4, of the periodic table of elements. Other elements in group 15 include nitrogen and phosphorous. Arsenic is another possible essential trace element. This may surprise some people who associate arsenic with poison.

It has been shown that minute traces of arsenic are in fact essential for certain animals. However, no clear biological function has been assigned to arsenic other than the observation that certain domestic animals appear to require it for thrifty growth. Studies have suggested that arsenic affects the formation of various metabolites of methionine including taurine and polyamines.
At one time, arsenic was used as a blanching agent to beautify the face and it was used therapeutically as a cure for syphilis.

The daily requirement for arsenic is unknown but the average daily intake is probable in the range 10 to 15 µg per day. The best sources of arsenic are shellfish, most meats especially liver. Many vegetables, including herbs, also contain traces of arsenic (from insecticides). Even water itself contains traces.

Arsenic is highly toxic and excessive intake may cause severe stomach and muscle pain, vomiting, diarrhoea, thirst, numbness and pins-and-needles. Chronic intake may first cause water-logging, inflammation of the eyelids and mouth, dermatitis, loss of hair and later it may lead to kidney, liver and brain damage with eventual death. A single dose of 100 mg arsenic in the form of arsenic trioxide can be fatal. The exact role of arsenic in humans, if any, is uncertain. A deficiency of arsenic in humans is unknown.

## Vanadium

Vanadium V, is a transition metal in the d-block, Group 5 (VA), Period 4, of the periodic table of elements.

Vanadium occurs in the blood cells of certain sea squirts and is also found in many terrestrial animals. Vanadium may exist in several chemical oxidation states. The vanadate anion, $VO_4^{3-}$, and the stable vanadyl or oxovanadium(IV) cation, $VO^{2+}$, are typical forms. Some possible functions of vanadium include the following. In certain marine species, it may act as an oxygen carrier in combination with a protein called vanadochrome. Vanadium has been found to have many *in vitro* and pharmacological actions.

Vanadium may inhibit the synthesis of cholesterol in the brain and thus lower the cholesterol level in the blood. This is possibly its most important regulatory function. It may also lower phospholipid levels in the blood and is therefore involved in many aspects of lipid metabolism. It may also be involved in blood production. It may act as a coenzyme in certain enzymes, particularly in lower microorganisms. And it may increase the contractile force of heart muscle. Vanadium stimulates the mineralization of bones and teeth and inhibits the development of dental caries in rats and guinea pigs.

It has been shown that vanadium can mimic the action of insulin in cell cultures, possibly by altering cell membrane function for ion transport processes and by making cell membrane insulin receptors more sensitive to insulin. Also, if diabetic rats are fed the vanadium salt, sodium metavanadate, in their drinking water, their blood glucose levels return to normal. Vanadium may help reduce the incidence of adult onset diabetes.

The daily requirement is unknown but an estimated 10 to 30 µg per day appears adequate. The best food sources include vegetables especially parsley, radishes, dill and lettuce, and sea food especially lobster, kelp and various fish (including bones as in sardines). certain processed foods may contain additional vanadium as a fortuitous contaminant. Stainless steel utensils used in cooking may also contribute significant amounts to the diet.

Vanadium is highly toxic and may cause a form of manic-depression in humans. Levels of intake over 5 milligrams per day are considered dangerous. Vitamin C in high doses combines with excess vanadium and may be used to detoxify such patients. In experimental studies with some animals, a deficiency of vanadium increased the lipid level in the blood including cholesterol. Deficiency may also cause anaemia and poor growth of bones and teeth. A deficiency of vanadium in humans is unknown.

**Gold**

Gold Au, is a metal in the d block, group 11 (1B), period 6, of the periodic table of elements. Group 11 also contains copper and silver.

Gold has no biological function. It interacts with proteins, amino acid residues and cell membrane receptors. Intramuscular injections (with a chemical compound containing gold called sodium aurothiomalate) have been used to dampen down some underlying rheumatic disease processes. It seems to reduce inflammation rather than simply treating the symptoms. However, gold also reduces the activity of the immune system and needs to be used carefully. It can decrease morning stiffness and pain and swelling in the joints. It is known as a disease-modifying antirheumatic drug.

# A4

## Common Toxicity and Deficiency Symptoms of Minerals and Trace Elements

**Table A4.1.i.** Minerals and trace elements

| NUTRIENT | TOXICITY | DEFICIENCY |
|---|---|---|
| **Minerals** | | |
| Potassium | Stomach ulcers. Renal failure. Cardiac arrest in diastole. | Acid-base disturbances, General weakness. Confusion. Heart attack. |
| Chloride | High blood pressure. Vomiting. Convulsions. Respiratory distress. Death. | Cramps, Apathy. Loss of appetite. Dehydration. Alkalosis. |
| Sodium | Thirst. Water retention. High blood pressure. Heart and kidney disease. Oedema. | Poor growth. Metabolic disturbances. Rapid heartbeat. Dehydration. Cramps. Poor appetite. |
| Calcium | Extremely rare, Phosphorous disturbances. Calcium deposition. Kidney stones. Inhibits absorption of other minerals. | Rickets in children. Osteomalacia in adults. Muscle pains. Lethargy. Tetany. |
| Phosphorous | Low blood calcium. Poor absorption of minerals. Deposition of calcium in tissues. | Extremely rare. Rickets in children. Osteomalacia in adults. Osteoporosis. |
| Magnesium | Diarrhoea. Low calcium. Depression of nervous system. Shallow breathing. | Generalised weakness. Cramps. Low blood pressure. Irritability. Tremor. Tetany. |

*Continued /*

**Table A4.1.ii.**

| NUTRIENT | TOXICITY | DEFICIENCY |
| --- | --- | --- |
| **Trace elements** | | |
| Iron | Haemosiderosis. Haemochromatosis. | Iron deficiency anaemia. Weakness. Poor resistance to infection. |
| Zinc | Zinc is relatively nontoxic. Copper, iron and other mineral imbalances. | Stunted growth dwarfism (nanism). Lack of sexual development. Poor appetite. Coarse skin. Poor wound healing. Susceptibility to infections. |
| Fluoride | Mottled teeth (Fluorosis). Dense bones (Osteosclerosis). Enzyme inhibition. | Increased tooth decay. |
| Manganese | Poor muscular coordination. Lethargy. Mental disturbances. | Enzyme disturbances. Possible growth disorders and poor sexual development. |
| **Ultratrace elements** | | |
| Copper | Nausea. Cramps. Cirrhosis of the liver. Kidney damage. | Microcytic anaemia. Brittle bones. Grey hair. Pale skin, Poor taste. |
| Iodine | May depress thyroid activity. Fever. Nausea. | Goitre. |
| Selenium | Bowel disorders. Irritable lungs. Garlic breath. Nervous disturbances. | Organ damage. Possible anaemia. Poor wound healing. Low vitamin E. |
| Molybdenum | Possible gout. Enzyme inhibition. Low copper. | Disturbances of sulphur metabolism. Low uric acid. |
| Chromium | Extremely rare. Organ damage. Lung cancer. Skin ulcers. | Diabetes. High cholesterol. Poor memory. Confusion. General malaise. |

# Bibliography

## General Reading

Bryce-Smyth, D. and Hodgkinson, L. (1986). The zinc solution, Century Arrow.

Burkitt, D. (1982). Don't forget the fibre in your diet, Third edition, Martin Dunitz.

Candlish, J. (1981). Metabolic water and the camel's hump—a textbook survey, *Biochemical Education* 9(3) 1981 96-97.

Cathie, K. (1976). The complete calorie counter, Pan Books.

Cathie, K. (1978). The complete carbohydrate counter, Pan Books.

Chaitow, L. (1985). Amino acids in therapy, Thorsons.

Forbes, A. (1990). Healthy eating: cooking with vitamins and minerals, Penguin Books.

Graham, J. and Odent, M. (1986). The Z factor, Thorsons.

Lewis, A. (1983). Selenium, Revised Expanded Edition Thorsons.

Mervyn, L. (1981). The B vitamins, Thorsons.

Mervyn, L. (1981). Vitamin C, Thorsons.

Mervyn, L. (1984). Vitamin E, Revised Edition, Nature's Way Series, Thorsons.

Mervyn, L. (1984). Vitamins A, D, K, Nature's Series, Thorsons.

Sherman, A. (1984). The sodium counter, Arlington Books.

Thomas, J. (1985). The fat counter, Pan Books.

Trimmer, E. (1987). The magic of magnesium, Thorsons.

Tudge, C. (1985). The food connection, BBC Publication.

Wright, M. (1984). The salt counter, Pan Books.

## Encyclopedias and Dictionaries

Adrian, J., Legrand, G and Frange, R. (1988). Dictionary of food and nutrition. Translator, B. Weitz. Translation Editors, E. Rolfe, I. Morton and L. Mabbit Ellis Horwood.

Black's agricultural dictionary, (1981). Edited by D. B. Dalal-Clayton Adam and Charles Black, Black Publishers Ltd.

Butterworth' s dictionary of nutrition and food technology, (1982). Edited by A. E. Bender, Butterworths.

Campion, K. (1986). Vegetarian encyclopedia, Century paperbacks.

Fischer, R. B. (1986). A dictionary of diets, slimming and nutrition, Paladin.

Illustrated Stedman's medical dictionary, (1982). 24th Edition, Williams and

Wilkins.

Kirschmann, J. D. (1979). Nutrition almanac, Revised Fourth Edition, McGraw-Hill.

Mayes, A. (1986). The dictionary of nutritional health: guide to the relation between diet and health, Thorsons.

McGraw-Hill Encyclopedia of food, agriculture and nutrition, (1977). Edited by D. N. Lapedes, McGraw-Hill.

Mervyn, L. (1986). Thorsons' complete guide to vitamins and minerals, Thorsons.

Scott, T. and Brewer, M. (1983). Concise encyclopedia of biochemistry, Walter de Gruyter.

Stenesh, J. (1975). Dictionary of biochemistry, John Wiley and Sons.

The encyclopedia of the biological sciences, (1983). Edited by P. Gray, Second Edition Van Nostrand.

Van Nostrand's scientific encyclopedia, (1983). Edited by D. M. Considine and G. D. Considine, Sixth Edition, Van Nostrand.

W. B. Saunders' atomic energy encyclopedia in the life sciences, (1964). Edited by C. Shilling, W. B. Saunders.

Yudkin, J. (1985). The penguin encyclopedia of nutrition, Penguin Books.

## Textbooks

Bell, G. H., Davison, J. N. and Emslie-Smyth, D. (1972). Textbook of physiology and biochemistry, Eight Edition, Churchill Livingstone.

Bohinski, H. C. (1979). Modern concepts in biochemistry, Third Edition, Allyn and Bacon.

Bowman, C. and Rand, M. J. (1980). Textbook of pharmacology, Second Edition, Blackwell Scientific Publications.

Burton, B. T. (1976). Human nutrition, Third Edition, McGraw-Hill.

Davidson and Passmore's human nutrition and dietetics, (1986). 8th Edition, Edited by R. Passmore and M. A. Eastwood, Churchill Livingstone.

Ganong, F. (1987). Review of medical physiology, Thirteenth Edition, Lange Medical Publications.

Gibney, M. J. (1986). Nutrition, diet and health, Cambridge University Press.

Goodman and Gillman's the pharmacological basis of therapeutics, (1985). Seventh Edition, Edited by A. G. Gilman, L. S. Goodman, T. W. Rall and F. Murad, Macmillan.

Green, J. H. (1980). An introduction to human physiology, Fourth (SI) Revised Edition, Oxford University Press.

Gurr, M. I. (1984). Role of fats in food and nutrition, Elsevier Applied

Science Publishers.

Gurr, M. I. and James, A. T. (1975). Lipid biochemistry, Second Edition, Chapman and Hall.

Guyton, A. C. (2006). Textbook of medical physiology, Eleventh Edition, W. B. Saunders.

Katzung, B. G. (Editor) (1984). Basic clinical pharmacology, 2nd Edition, Lange Medical Publications.

Lehninger, A. L. (1982). Principles of Biochemistry, Worth Publishers Inc.

Lloyde, L. E., McDonald, B. E. and Crampton, E. W. (1978). Fundamentals of nutrition, Second Edition, W. H. Freeman and Co.

McDonald, P., Edwards, R. A. and Greenhalgh, J. F. D. (1988). Animal nutrition, Longman, Scientific and Technical.

Metzler, D. E. (1977). Biochemistry: the chemical reactions of living cells, Academic Press.

Murray, R. K., Granner, D. K., Mayes, P. A. and Rodwell, V. W. (1990). Harper's biochemistry, Twenty-Second Edition, Lange Medical Books.

Ottaway, J. H. and Apps, D. K. (1984). Biochemistry, Fourth Edition, Baillière Tyndall.

Peterson, C. R. (1983). Essentials of human biochemistry, Pitman Books.

Smith, E. L., Hill, R. L., Lehman, I. R., Lefkowitz, R. J., Handler, P. and White, A. (1983). Principles of biochemistry: mammalian biochemistry, Seventh Edition McGraw-Hill.

Taylor, T. G. (1978). Principles of human nutrition, The Institute of Biology Series No 94, Edward Arnold.

Vander, A. J., Sherman, J. H. and Luciane, D. S. (1984). Human physiology: the mechanism of body function, Fourth Edition, McGraw-Hill.

Wills, E. D. (1985). Biochemical basis of medicine, John Wright and Sons.

## Reference Works

Assmann, G. (1982). Lipid metabolism and atherosclerosis, F. K. Schattauer Verlag.

Bender, A. E. and Bender, D. A. (1986). Food tables, Oxford University Press.

Biochemical nomenclature and related documents, (1978). International Union of Biochemistry, as reprinted for the Biochemical Society by Spottiswoode Ballantyne Press.

Biological handbooks (new series) Vol II: Human health and disease, (1977). Edited by P. L. Altman and D. Dittmer Katz, Fed. Amer. Soc. Exp. Biol., Bethesda, Maryland.

Biological handbooks: blood and other body fluids (1961). Edited by P. L. Altman and D. S. Dittmer, Fed. Amer. Soc. Exp. Biol., Bethesda, Maryland.

Biological handbooks: metabolism, (1968). Edited by P. L. Altman and D. S. Dittmer, Fed. Amer. Soc. Exp. Biol., Bethesda, Maryland.

CRC handbook of biochemistry: selected data for molecular biology, (1970). 2nd Edition, Edited by H. A. Sober, CRC Press.

CRC handbook of chemistry and physics, (1981). 62nd Edition, Edited by R. C. Weast and M. J. Astle, CRC Press.

CRC handbook of eicosanoids: prostaglandins and related lipids, Vol I (Part A): Biochemical aspects (1987). Edited by A. L. Willis, CRC Press.

CRC handbook series. Nutrition and food: Section E, nutritional disorders, Vol I. Effects of nutrient excesses and toxicities in animals and man, (1977). Edited by M. Rechcigl, Jr., CRC Press.

Food and agriculture organisation: energy yielding components of food and computation of caloric values. (1947). F.A.O. Nutrition Division.

Food, nutrition and climate (1982). Edited by K. Blaxter and L. Fowden, Applied Science Publishers.

Geigy Scientific Tables: Eight revised and enlarged edition, Edited by C. Lentner, Ciba-Geigy.

Handbook of vitamins: nutritional, biochemical and clinical aspects (1984). Edited by L. J. Machlin, Marcel Dekker.

Nutrient interactions, (1988). Edited by C. E. Bodwell and J. W. Erdman, Jr., Marcel Dekker.

Osborne, D. R. and Voogt, P. (1978). The analysis of nutrients in foods, Academic Press.

Paul, A. A. and Southgate, D. A. T. (1978). McCance and Widdowson's the composition of foods, Fourth Edition, H. M. Stationary Office London.

Paul, A. A., Southgate, D. A. T., and Russell, J. (1980). First supplement to McCance and Widdowson's the composition of foods, H. M. Stationary Office London.

Reeds, P. J., (2000). "Dispensable and indispensable amino acids for humans", *American Society for Nutritional Sciences, Supplement.* 1835S–1840S.

Recommended dietary allowances (1989). Tenth Edition, Food and Nutrition Board, National Academy of Sciences - National Research Council, US.

Requirements of vitamin A, iron, folate and vitamin B12 (1988). Report of joint FAO/WHO expert consultation. Food and Agriculture Organisation of the United Nations, Rome.

Shamberger, R. J. (1983). Biochemistry of the elements: Vol 2. Biochemistry of selenium, Plenum Press.

Trace elements in human and animal nutrition: Vol 2 (1986). Fifth Edition, Edited by W. Mertz, Orlando, Academic Press.

Van Dorp, P. A. (1973). Essential fatty acids and prostaglandins: Vol 2. Butterworths.

World Health Organisation: handbook on human nutritional requirements (1974). Monograph Series No. 61, WHO in collaboration with the Food and Agriculture Organisation of the United Nations.

## Web Sources

Dietary Reference Intakes, (1997 – 2011). National Academies Press.

Dietary Reference Intakes for Calcium, Phosphorous, Magnesium, Vitamin D, and Fluoride (1997);

Dietary Reference Intakes for Thiamin, Riboflavin, Niacin, Vitamin B6, Folate, Vitamin B12, Pantothenic Acid, Biotin, and Choline (1998);

Dietary Reference Intakes for Vitamin C, Vitamin E, Selenium, and Carotenoids (2000);

Dietary Reference Intakes for Vitamin A, Vitamin K, Arsenic, Boron, Chromium, Copper, Iodine, Iron, Manganese, Molybdenum, Nickel, Silicon, Vanadium, and Zinc (2001);

Dietary Reference Intakes for Energy, Carbohydrate, Fiber, Fat, Fatty Acids, Cholesterol, Protein, and Amino Acids (2002/2005);

Dietary Reference Intakes for Calcium and Vitamin D (2011);

Note: These reports may be accessed via: *www.nap.edu.*

Dietary Reference Intakes (DRIs): Estimated Average Requirements. Food and Nutrition Board, Institute of Medicine, National Academies. Life Stage. Group. *https://fnic.nal.usda.gov/sites/fnic.nal.usda.gov/files/uploads/recommended_ intakes_individuals.pdf* [modified: 16 December 2015].

Greene, W., (2016). DC Nutrition.com, Minerals, *http://www.dcnutrition.com/minerals/minerals.cfm* [retrieved, 18 December 2016].
Dr Greene's website is a concise summary of information on all trace elements and other nutrients.

United States Department of Agriculture, National Agricultural Library (USDA, NAL), DRI Tables and Application Reports, *https://fnic.nal.usda.gov/dietary-guidance/dietary-reference-intakes* [modified: 30 April 2016].
*https://fnic.nal.usda.gov/dietary-guidance/dietary-reference-intakes/ dri-tables-and-application-reports* [retrieved: 28 September 2016].

Dietary Reference Intakes (DRIs) are developed and published by the Institute of Medicine (IOM). The DRIs represent the most current scientific knowledge on nutrient needs of healthy populations.

Dietary Reference Intakes for Energy, Carbohydrate, Fiber, Fat, Fatty Acids, Cholesterol, Protein, and Amino Acids (Macronutrients), (2005). National Academies Press. *http://www.nap.edu/catalog/10490/ dietary-reference-intakes-for-energy-carbohydrate-fiber-fat-fatty-acids-cholesterol-protein-and-amino-acids-macronutrients* [modified: 7 April 2016].

Health Supplements & Nutritional Health. *http://www.healthsupplementsnutritionalguide.com/* [retrieved: 14 January 2017].

Linus Pauling Institute, Micronutrient Information Center. Oregon State University. Choline, *http://lpi.oregonstate.edu/mic/other-nutrients/choline* [retrieved: 29 April 2016].

Linus Pauling Institute, Micronutrient Information Center. Oregon State University. Essential Fatty Acids, *http://lpi.oregonstate.edu/mic/other-nutrients/essential-fatty-acids* [retrieved: 28 September 2016].

The Linus Pauling Institute is a valuable authoritative source of information on the nutrients.
Nielsen, F.H. Ultratrace elements. Chapter 33, pp 401 – 415. *https://naldc.nal.usda.gov/download/48282/PDF* [retrieved: 18 January 2017].

Nielsen, F.H. Other trace elements. Chapter 35, pp 354–377. *https://naldc.nal.usda.gov/download/45343/PDF* [retrieved: 22 January 2017].

Dr Forrest H. Nielsen has carried out Trojan work on the Ultratrace Elements in Nutrition.
Payne, P.R., (1971). Reference protein patterns, 1–8, *ftp://ftp.fao.org/docrep/fao/meeting/009/ae906e/ae906e25.pdf* [modified: 12 October 2016].

Rouzer, C.A. (2014). Bromide ion is essential for life, The Vanderbilt Institute of Chemical Biology. *http://www.vanderbilt.edu/vicb/DiscoveriesArchives/bromide_ion_essential_life.html* [modified 22 September 2014].

Supplements-And-Health.com. (2016). Lesser Known Facts About Tryptophan Side Effects. *http://www.supplements-and-health.com/tryptophan-side-effects.html* [retrieved: 21 October 2016].

University of Maryland Medical Centre. (2016). Phenylalanine, *http://umm.edu/health/medical/altmed/supplement/phenylalanine* [retrieved:

17 October 2016].

US Department of Agriculture, National Agricultural Library. (2016). DRI Nutrient Reports. *https://fnic.nal.usda.gov/dietary-guidance/dietary-reference-intakes/dri-nutrient-reports* [retrieved, 18 October 2016].

Uthman, E. (2007). Elemental composition of the human body. *http://web2.airmail.net/uthman/elements_of_body.html* [modified: 15 May 2007].

Wikipedia (2017). Composition of the human body, *https://en.wikipedia.org/wiki/Composition_of_the_human_body#Elemental_composition_list* [modified: 14 January 2017].

Wikipedia. (2016). "Essential amino acid", *https://en.wikipedia.org/wiki/Essential_amino_acid* [modified: 11 October 2016].

# About the Author

### Richard Rydon

Richard Rydon is an award-winning science fiction novelist. His three books in the Luper Series, The Oortian Summer (2007), The Omega Wave (2008) and The Palomar Paradox: A SETI Mystery (2011), have been given excellent reviews.

Richard's second novel, The Omega Wave, was selected as one of the finalists in the Science Fiction Category of the Reader Views Literary Awards and was awarded an Honorary Mention (Third Place) in the Reviewers Choice Awards in 2009.

His third novel, The Palomar Paradox, won the Bronze/3rd Place award in the Romance Category of the Feathered Quill Book Awards in 2014.

Richard is an honours science graduate. He has also obtained numerous certificates and diplomas in Psychology, Counselling, Theology, and a Diplôme de Cuisine Française. He is a prolific writer and has published over 300 papers, articles and poems, in scientific journals, magazines and local papers to date.

He has also published a second edition of his anthology of poetry, titled A Golden Fuchsia-Laden Girl (2011), containing 100 poems.

### About the Science Fiction Novels in the Luper Series

*The Oortian Summer*

'The Oortian Summer' is a romantic science fiction adventure involving co-worker relationships in an astronomical observatory as two massive comets approach the Earth. The unusual twist in the story involves a perilous attempt, proposed by Luper, the lead character, to bring the comets even closer to Earth to prevent a catastrophic geomagnetic flip.

*The Omega Wave*

'The Omega Wave' is a gothic science fiction novel. Aided and

114

abetted by Quade their boss, Luper and Frieda progress secretly and meticulously, to develop biological computers called neurospheres. Working in the shadow of a rogue American Embassy, they first conceal but later reveal what they have seen and done.

### *The Palomar Paradox: A SETI Mystery*

'The Palomar Paradox' sees Luper back in an astronomical observatory searching for signs of extraterrestrial intelligence. He finds himself working with Leila, a young girl recovering from leukaemia, and Karina, an experienced astronomer, among others. As their research continues, unusual signals are picked up by their radio telescope. The signals are explained, one by one, until ... !

## About Richard Rydon's Poetry

### *A Golden Fuchsia-Laden Girl*

'A Golden Fuchsia-Laden Girl' is an anthology of one hundred poems of whimsy, innocence and longing, by Richard Rydon, written and revised between 1957 and 2011. Twenty poems have been added in this second edition.

## About Richard Rydon's Non-Fiction Books

### *Matter, Energy and Mentality: Exploring Metaphysical Reality*

His non-fiction book, 'Matter, Energy and Mentality: Exploring Metaphysical Reality', was published in 2012. 'Matter, Energy and Mentality' is a book of speculative non-fiction. It covers the relationships between Matter, Energy and Mentality, using Energy Redistribution (Unnecessary Action) as a common feature in the Universe.

### *Profiles of the Nutrients*

'Profiles of the Nutrients — 1. Carbohydrate, Lipid, and Protein' published in 2016, is the first book in a series about the nutrients which are essential for human life.

The other books in the series are titled as follows:

'Profiles of the Nutrients — 2. Minerals and Trace Elements'.
'Profiles of the Nutrients — 3. Water-Soluble and Fat-Soluble
Vitamins'.

www.ingramcontent.com/pod-product-compliance
Lightning Source LLC
Chambersburg PA
CBHW060406290526
45791CB00002B/626